Post-Pregnancy
PILATES

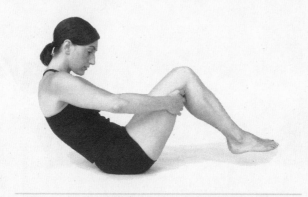

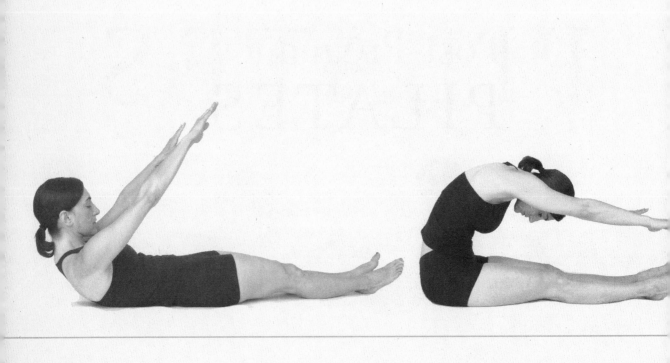

AVERY
a member of
Penguin Group (USA) Inc.
New York
2005

Post-Pregnancy
PILATES

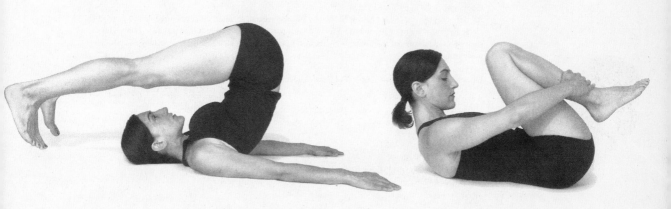

AN ESSENTIAL GUIDE FOR A FIT BODY AFTER BABY

Karrie Adamany

Published by the Penguin Group

Penguin Group (USA) Inc., 375 Hudson Street, New York, New York 10014, USA · Penguin Group (Canada), 10 Alcorn Avenue, Toronto, Ontario M4V 3B2, Canada (a division of Pearson Penguin Canada Inc.) · Penguin Books Ltd, 80 Strand, London WC2R 0RL, England · Penguin Ireland, 25 St Stephen's Green, Dublin 2, Ireland (a division of Penguin Books Ltd) · Penguin Group (Australia), 250 Camberwell Road, Camberwell, Victoria 3124, Australia (a division of Pearson Australia Group Pty Ltd) · Penguin Books India Pvt Ltd, 11 Community Centre, Panchsheel Park, New Delhi–110 017, India · Penguin Group (NZ), Cnr Airborne and Rosedale Roads, Albany, Auckland 1310, New Zealand (a division of Pearson New Zealand Ltd) · Penguin Books (South Africa) (Pty) Ltd, 24 Sturdee Avenue, Rosebank, Johannesburg 2196, South Africa · Penguin Books Ltd, Registered Offices: 80 Strand, London WC2R 0RL, England

Library of Congress Cataloging-in-Publication Data

Adamany, Karrie.
    Post-pregnancy Pilates : an essential guide for a fit body after baby / Karrie
Adamany.
        p.   cm.
    Includes index.
    ISBN 1-58333-226-X
    1. Pilates method.   2. Exercise for women.   3. Physical fitness for women.
4. Mothers—Health and hygiene.   5. Postnatal care.   I. Title.
RA781.4.A33   2005   2004062314
613.7'045—dc22

Printed in the United States of America
10 9 8 7 6 5 4 3 2 1

BOOK DESIGN BY DEBORAH KERNER DESIGN
INTERIOR PHOTOGRAPHS BY SHANNON FAGAN

Most Avery books are available at special quantity discounts for bulk purchase for sales promotions, premiums, fund-raising, and educational needs. Special books or book excerpts also can be created to fit specific needs. For details, write Penguin Group (USA) Inc. Special Markets, 375 Hudson Street, New York, NY 10014.

ACKNOWLEDGMENTS

I would like to thank Kirsten Manges for her persistence and patience, my friends for their endless encouragement and proofreadings, and my family—especially my mother and three sisters—for their support and amazing Chester-sitting capabilities. For assistance on this book, thanks go to Sarah Reed (the student and the teacher); Wendy Quitasol; Deborah Goldfrank, OB/GYN; Shannon Fagan (photographer); and Mako Iijima and Hiro Yonemoto (hair and makeup). Special thanks to my girls, including Melissa M., Melissa B., Andrea, Linda, Maya, Patricia, Lina, Liz, Lee, Tania, Pixie, Alina, Ambrosia, Mandy, Nicki, Frances, Rochelle, Susan, Joan, Katie, Micky, Sloane, Jan, Sally, Sherry, Susana, Maritzha, Nicole, Jenna, Jackie, Rose, and my editor, Kristen Jennings. My biggest thanks go to Mark Pollard, for co-creating the most amazing being in the world, Chester.

CONTENTS

Post-Pregnancy
PILATES

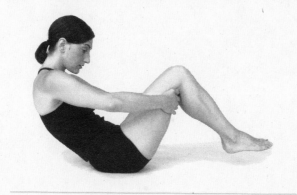

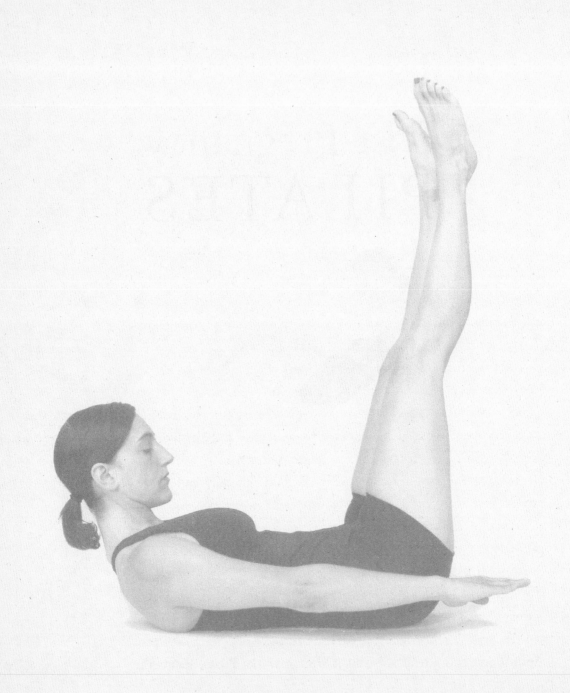

INTRODUCTION

Presumably, you have already experienced one of the wonders of being a woman: giving birth to your child. Now reward yourself with a gift that will help you cope with the state of your body and your new life. *Post-Pregnancy Pilates* will help you address your physical postpartum predicament and enjoy your baby by showing you how to appreciate and accept your new body and self. With Pilates you can regain your strength and your pre-pregnancy body—or improve it.

Women are inherently strong. That's why we have the babies! We often do not acknowledge or realize our own strength that enables us to raise children, have a career, take care of our families and home, etc. We are just expected (by ourselves and by others) to get the job done. But what is strength and where does it come from? You must be strong to carry a child—literally and figuratively. You carry the baby throughout your pregnancy, you carry the toddler until he is too heavy to lift any longer, and you carry the child emotionally until adulthood. The point is you need to be strong. Strong in every way.

So why is Pilates better than anything else to help build the strength mothers need? Why should you do Pilates rather than go to the gym, hire a trainer, or go back to your pre-pregnancy routine, if you had one at all? This is why: it works. Pilates meets the postpartum body reshaping challenge head-on. Say good-bye to your fatigued and flabby figure because with *Post-Pregnancy Pilates* you will:

- recover from the physical pain and strain of childbirth,
- get rid of your post-pregnancy belly and added weight,
- become more toned and fit than you were before you had your baby,
- build physical strength and mental stamina,
- gain vital energy you will need to keep up with your new little one,
- change the way you stand, sit, sleep, enjoy sex, walk, and carry things, all the while protecting you from injuring your already weary body.

And best of all, it is time- and cost-effective. It takes only a few minutes per day in your own home and without equipment.

I have experienced all the benefits of Pilates myself after the birth of my son, Chester. Before Ches was born, I had always been active and exercised in some form or another, whether it was scampering about in a hideous plaid skirt on the field hockey team, running on a treadmill, or lifting weights next to muscle heads at the gym. But after giving birth I was weak and droopy and flat. I thought I was doomed to be dumpy. Then a friend gave me a gift certificate for a Pilates lesson. I had read about Pilates and the celebrities and models who raved about it, but I still had no idea what it was all about. During the first lesson, as I sat on the equipment looking in the mirror at my profile, I didn't know if I wanted to laugh or cry. My instructor was tall and lovely with just the right amount of muscle, wearing form-fitting pants and a tiny T-shirt, and I was soft and flabby with baggy clothes that could not hide my gigantic nursing breasts. It was mortifying. Sure I loved my son, and I missed him desperately for that hour and a half I was away from him, but he was responsible for this mess that was my body. And to make matters worse, as I followed her instructions, it was as though I was learning how to move my body for the first time. It felt like a cruel joke.

But despite the humiliation of that moment in the mirror, I kept going back for more. And I saw results I never expected. My body shape began to transform after just a few weeks and I felt great! Pilates gave me energy, unlike other exercise I had done, which normally depleted my energy. My body looked fantastic— much better than it did before I became pregnant—and my brain was happy from being challenged by the focus and coordination required to do the movements. I developed core strength and completely changed the shape of my body. Pilates toned my muscles (making them lean but not bulky), slimmed my hips, lifted my butt, sculpted my arms and legs, and gave me six-pack abs that crunches never could. Pilates had such an impact on my health and fitness that I decided to become an instructor.

The program that I developed for new mothers takes into account all the lessons I learned from my own pregnancy and recovery experience. Now, in *Post-Pregnancy Pilates*, new mothers can discover a fitness program that focuses on the muscle groups that are stressed during pregnancy and delivery and on postural alignment and stability, which has been compromised by the shifting of your center of gravity during the prenatal period. In this book, I do not cover the entire Pilates method, but instead offer workouts that begin by gently invigorating and healing your postpartum body. Gradually, the workouts increase in difficulty and intensity and will help you lose weight, firm your muscles, and build core strength and stability in order to give you the body you deserve.

This method provides solutions to common physical obstacles women find while recovering from, let's be honest here, the bodily destruction incurred during pregnancy and childbirth. Pilates can also help to decrease fatigue, back pain, constipation, weight retention, anxiety, and depression, and will improve your strength and endurance, energy level, posture, circulation, general sense of well-being, and most important, your recovery time after delivery.

I like to think of it as building self-confidence through self-improvement. Through Pilates, I improved my self-esteem by feeling better about my physical self. You too can gain mental clarity when you focus on strengthening your physical self and concentrate on truly feeling the power of these movements. Focus is what makes Pilates, and *Post-Pregnancy Pilates*, all about you.

Pilates is about finding balance in your life. As a mother, every hour of the day is accounted for before you get out of bed, so your time—and time for you—is more precious than ever. I hope you will use this book to focus your mind and body—and to tap into your inner strength and discover how much more wonderful motherhood can be when you make time for yourself.

1

Getting Started

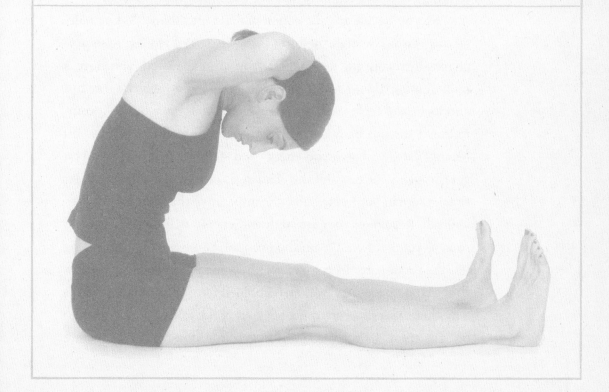

The main complaint I hear from postpartum women—besides that they are overwhelmingly fatigued—is that their bodies are ruined. Gone. Destroyed. The worst moment for me was seeing a photo of my son in my arms in the hospital. His sweet little face, his delicate fingers, thick messy hair, tiny head, and . . . what was that giant flesh pillow he was resting on? Was it—horror—my giant flabby arm? Upon further scrutiny, I realized it was a mammoth breast. Scary just the same. It made me feel huge and awkward and like a troll next to my beautiful little baby. But this is not just vanity. Think about it. You want to be yourself, the "you" that you formerly knew. You want to be desirable to your partner again. You are tired of wearing maternity clothes and stretched-out sweatpants.

So you decide to take action and get into shape. But actually getting started is often the most difficult part of any exercise program—especially for new moms. You are exhausted, you have a million other things to do, and your body is not only weaker but also looks and feels, well, different. But if you make health a commitment to your baby and yourself, you will feel better once you begin. Pilates will give you energy and strength that will help you get through your day and the challenges of raising a child. In order to take care of your new baby it is imperative that you take care of yourself. Regaining your strength and energy will be important as soon as you get home from the hospital. You will likely be getting less than adequate sleep, no matter how many catnaps you are able to sneak in. Sleep deprivation, combined with your innate sense as a mother to sacrifice anything for your child, causes the body to go on "autopilot" to get through the day. You don't have to operate this way. In my case, I took advantage of my husband and girl-friends in the early months. Being able to hand off the baby to go exercise or even to run errands made a huge difference to my disposition.

Although your number-one priority is your baby, my message to you is that you must still take time for yourself. We all need a little respite now and then, but making the best use of your alone time—and making sure you create some alone time—is truly self-preservation. The best thing about the *Post-Pregnancy Pilates* program is that you don't even have to leave home to exercise. When the baby is napping or your friends are over to admire the little one, go to a room and close the door to exercise and take time for yourself. Pilates can help you balance your mind and your body. Just give yourself a moment of quiet to remember yourself amid the maelstrom of motherhood.

Before beginning your Pilates program, try to keep in mind a few basics in order to prepare your body. First, you must consult with your doctor before you begin an exercise program. Second, eating right will help you to stay healthy during this transitional time for your body. And third, any seasoned mother will tell you that you must never sacrifice sleep for housework or other such trivialities!

Now it is time to begin. In this chapter, you will learn how to engage your abdominal muscles and you will be introduced to the Baby Steps Workout. This routine, done as a whole or broken down as individual exercises, is the first step to your recovery. Each exercise or stretch will get you gently moving and bring you closer to your goal of becoming a fit mom.

ADVICE FOR
NURSING MOTHERS

Breast-feeding affects the kinds of exercises you can do right away. Your breasts will be even bigger than they were during pregnancy. For example, I went from a 34D pre-pregnancy, to a 36DD during pregnancy, to a 38E right after I gave birth. My friends were shocked and amazed. Thankfully, I finally went down to a more manageable size after several weeks, because those girls were downright scary. The increased size of your breasts affects your posture and can create stress on your spine, and your breasts will be sore and most likely engorged a few days after delivery.

Doing exercises on your stomach may be uncomfortable, but you are by now accustomed to lying on your side and back. To reduce the weight of your breasts, you should nurse before exercising. Wear a supportive bra that is not too tight, and be ready for some surprises. A couple of months postpartum I decided to try a neighborhood yoga class, excited to have some time for myself. Ten minutes into the class I was apparently so relaxed that my breasts started to leak. Noticeably leak. I was too embarrassed to stay. But if I had had some of those nifty breast pads I would have been downward dogging happily. So *be prepared for anything*. In fact, this should be your new Mommy Mantra.

Correct Your Posture

One of the first steps to recovery is realigning your posture. Despite the fact that you may not be able to locate any of your abdominal muscles at this point, you need to begin to be aware of your posture (which comes from your abs) while sitting, standing, feeding your baby, bending over to pick him up, changing diapers, etc. Practicing good posture will enable you to lug around all your new motherly accessories. You will read "engage your abdominal muscles" over and over again in this book. By engage, I mean contract, or "lift," your abdominal muscles by pulling them in and up. This action isolates your abs without sticking out your ribs or jutting out your chest. Be sure to practice easy breathing while engaging these muscles, as holding your breath creates tension in your body. Practice isolating your abs as you move around your house. Once you get the hang of this contraction, it will become second nature to use your abdominal muscles in daily activities.

Identify Who You Are

The kind of delivery you had and your doctor's recommendations will determine when you can start an exercise program. However, most people can begin doing small movements immediately after giving birth that will actually accelerate the recovery process.

If you had a vaginal delivery, chances are you also had an episiotomy, or at least a small tear. This was the most painful part of the recovery process for me. The most clever invention ever, in my opinion, is the ice pack disguised as a maxi pad. It provided the ultimate relief. The problem was that I couldn't take any home with me. And after one week at home the pain was so excruciating that I went back to my doctor convinced that something was wrong with me, even though I wasn't scheduled to go in for another week. I was fine, healing normally . . . just being completely wimpy. And after another week the pain was gone.

If you had a C-section, you need not worry about the pain down under. It is the tingling, numbness, or prickly feeling around the scar that will concern you. Although a cesarean section is surgery, remember that your muscles (wherever they are) are still, in most cases, intact. You will likely be sensitive in the lower abdominal area and should take care of the scar as you would any other. You should be ready to do the exercises on the following pages shortly after delivery. If you feel any discomfort or swelling around your scar, allow yourself a little extra time to heal and talk to your doctor before taking on deeper abdominal work.

Rediscover Your Abdominal Muscles

Diastasis recti, or separations of the recti muscles, are fairly common during pregnancy. These abdominal muscles that normally run parallel lengthwise must expand and stretch away from your midline to allow more space for your growing baby. To check for separation, lie on your back with your knees bent and feet on the floor. Place two fingers just below your navel and apply gentle pressure to your abdomen while engaging your abdominal muscles. Begin to slowly lift your head and shoulders off the floor while maintaining pressure with your fingers. As you lift your head and shoulders, it should feel as though the two bands of recti muscles are closing in around your fingers. If you cannot feel this, try to curl your head and shoulders up a little farther.

If you find that your abdominal muscles are separated more than two fingers wide, don't panic—you will still be able to recover your abdominal strength. You will, however, need to be more aware of bulging that can occur while exercising. In other words, if you notice a small abdominal bubble expanding while exercising, stop and/or modify your movement. The C-section modification, which will provide more explicit instructions on how to watch out for and correct this, will follow in the exercise section.

Whether you had a vaginal or C-section delivery, to ensure that you heal properly, you need to strengthen and shorten the abdominal muscles that have been stretched. It is important to remember that while you do postpartum Pilates exercises you should always have your abdominal muscles engaged and pulled in. In the Baby Steps Workout (page 15), the Pelvic Curl exercise will help you rediscover your abdominal muscles through gentle contracting exercises. If you feel pain or detect your diastasis recti are actually separating more, you should contact your physician to get hands-on help.

Zero in on Back Pain

Many women experience back pain during pregnancy, which is caused by the changes our bodies go through in order to make room for the growing baby. The softening of ligaments surrounding your joints, especially in the pelvis, hips, and lower spine, decreases stability in this area. Your growing belly also causes a shift forward in your pelvis that creates a curve (swayback) in your lower spine. In addition, to compensate for the swaying lower back, your chest and shoulders are pulled forward and inward. And as your abdominal wall is stretched and weakened, the lower back muscles bear much of the load and the upper back and chest muscles elongate and tighten. Weight gain and joint laxity can also cause damage to your knees by hyperextending them, as well as weak and/or swollen ankles and dropped arches in your feet. All of this, combined with the extra weight you are carrying in the front of your body, can result in back pain, muscular imbalances, and quite possibly some beautiful shoes that no longer fit.

To zero in on this postpartum predicament, you must work first and foremost on the pelvic floor muscles. It is very important to re-tone these muscles after vaginal delivery, and especially before jumping into any form of exercise. These muscles support your organs, dictate urinary control, and counter increased pressure from actions such as sneezing, coughing, jumping, running, etc. And of course toned pelvic floor muscles can increase sexual pleasure for both parties.

If you had a cesarean delivery, you are not off the hook. Pressure from pushing during labor can stretch the pelvic floor, and just the increased weight of carrying the baby for nine months can do a number on these muscles.

The Baby Steps Workout (page 15) starts you off with Kegel exercises to work on the pelvic floor muscles. Don't be surprised if you cannot feel significant movement of the pelvic floor. With practice these muscles will strengthen and you will gain better control of the muscle contraction. Much like doing Pilates, Kegel exercises require focus, and with practice you will gain muscle memory and feel a deeper connection to the muscles.

What to Wear

You should wear comfortable clothing that allows for easy movement, but don't hide your body. You may not like what you see today, but it is helpful to see your body moving to make sure you are doing the exercises correctly.

Where to Exercise

You can do Pilates almost anywhere, as long as you have enough space to move your body freely on and around your exercise surface. You can begin by working out on a towel, but I recommend that you eventually invest in an exercise mat as well as 2- to 3-pound weights. A mat will provide more support than a towel on the floor, and small weights are inexpensive and easy to store.

Tip: Every new day is a new opportunity for you to do one thing for yourself. You'll feel better for it, and will end up with more to give to your baby.

2

The Baby Steps Workout

WEEKS 1–2

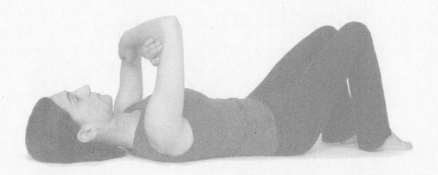

You may never be more tired in your life than you are in the days after you have your baby. It's not your standard didn't-get-enough-sleep tired, but rather a combination of physical exhaustion from the birth itself and the all-consuming mental and emotional enthusiasm directed at your new baby. I felt like a zombie sleepwalking through the first few days after Ches was born, not knowing what time of day it was or even what day of the week. My baby was attached to me as we moved from the bed to the kitchen to the couch. When I was able to muster up enough energy to get down on the floor with him, stretching and gentle abdominal exercises felt great and helped me out of my postpartum brain fog.

The truth is that you won't feel like doing much more than holding your bundle of joy or sleeping. But the movements in this chapter will gently invigorate your muscles, make you more alert, relieve stiffness or tension in your body, and help you to get a more restful sleep—all of which will help your physical recovery from childbirth.

Tip: Have a sense of humor about your condition. Laughing is good exercise.

The Baby Steps Workout includes exercises that you can do while still in the hospital that will wake up parts of your body you had forgotten about in the past months. These exercises and stretches will help you to start moving and will alleviate stress and stiffness caused by lying in your hospital bed and staring at the less-than-appetizing food. For the first two weeks after giving birth I recommend you do this workout fifteen minutes each day, or as long as it takes you to get through this short series, but don't stop there. You can continue to incorporate these exercises into your program for a few weeks and then use them as needed indefinitely. Remember to start slowly, increasing the duration and intensity of your workout gradually. Also, be sure to hydrate, hydrate, hydrate! You must drink lots of water all day long, and especially while exercising. This is particularly important if you are breastfeeding.

While doing these and all the exercises in this book, keep in mind the goals of *Post-Pregnancy Pilates*:

- to strengthen the body, especially the abdominal and pelvic floor muscles (core muscles), which suffered the most damage during pregnancy;
- to realign the body;
- to promote awareness of the extra flexibility that remains in the joints, and will remain for some time, especially if you are breastfeeding.

17

Kegel *(Pelvic Floor Lift)*

PURPOSE: **Strengthen the pelvic floor; facilitate recovery of the perineal area.**

The mother of all exercises, this one should be done before, during, and after pregnancy. In fact, Kegel exercises are the one exercise that every woman needs. They work the pelvic floor muscles that support your internal organs, which really take a beating during pregnancy. Kegel exercises can be done sitting, standing, lying down, in a car, on an elevator, watching TV, or during a particularly boring phone conversation.

Contract (lift) and tighten your pelvic floor muscles by pulling them in and up. A common way to describe this action is to utilize the muscles that would stop a urine stream. Hold for five counts then release while breathing normally, trying to isolate these muscles without engaging your abdominals or buttocks. As you contract the pelvic floor your belly should flatten. Do a set of five repetitions at first, then when you are stronger, increase the repetitions and the amount of time that you hold for ten counts. You can never do enough of these, so if you are really diligent do a few sets throughout the day. You can incorporate this exercise with other Pilates exercises, which will be noted later in the book.

The most common mistakes made during pelvic floor exercises include holding the breath, bearing down (the opposite of what you are trying to accomplish), and tensing the upper abdominal muscles and buttocks.

Breathing Exercise

PURPOSE: **Relaxation, circulation, and focus.**

Lying flat on your back, bend your knees and keep your feet on the ground, hip-distance apart. Place your hands lightly on your ribs with your fingertips barely touching and take a deep breath in through the nose, feeling your lungs and ribs expand. Exhale through the mouth, releasing all the air, feeling your ribs (and fingertips) come back together. Repeat five times.

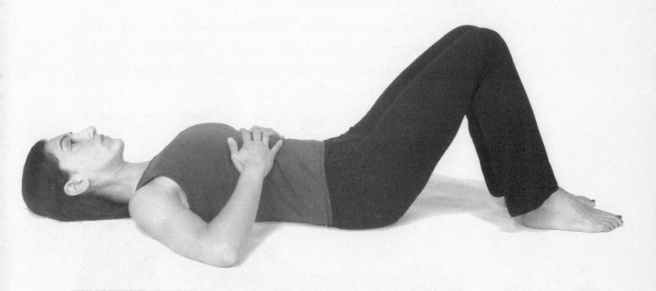

Breathing Exercise

Pelvic Curl

PURPOSE: **Release tension in the lower back by lengthening the spine; strengthen the abdominal muscles and pelvic floor.**

Lying flat on your back, bend your knees and keep your feet on the ground, hip-distance apart. Completely relax your upper body, reaching your shoulder blades down your back. Engage (or imagine engaging) your lower abdominal muscles by pulling them in. This subtle movement will result in your tailbone reaching away from your body and your spine lengthening.

Hold for ten counts. Release slowly without creating tension in your upper back. Repeat three times in the beginning, working your way up to five, and later ten. Be sure to breathe normally. When you have mastered the Pelvic Curl, add a Kegel (page 18) while you hold the curl. Release the Kegel hold as you release the curl position.

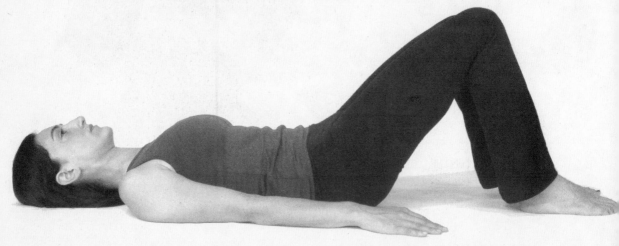

Pelvic Curl

Spine Release

PURPOSE: Release tension in the lower back and stretch the back of the thighs.

Lying flat on your back, bend your knees and keep your feet flat on the ground, hip-distance apart. Keep your entire spine touching the mat, floor, or bed by pulling your abdominal muscles in. Bring your knees into your chest and place your hands under the back of your thighs. Inhale, pull the knees in closer to your chest and allow your spine to lengthen, keeping your tailbone down. Exhale and relax into the position. Hold for ten counts. Continue to breathe normally while holding the stretch. Repeat as necessary. Make sure that you keep your head down and relaxed during this stretch.

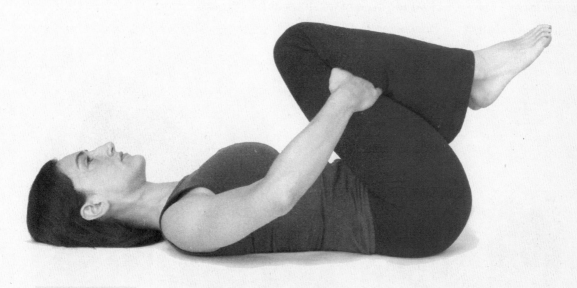

Spine Release

Shoulder Stretch Reclined

PURPOSE: Strengthen the upper back, release tension in the shoulders, and strengthen the abdominal muscles.

Lying on your back, bend your knees and place your feet flat on the floor, hip-distance apart. Clasp your elbows with opposite hands, your arms crossing parallel to your chest. Keeping your shoulders down on the mat, engage your abdominal muscles and press your back into the floor. Your tailbone should stay on the mat, reaching long. Without arching your back, pull your shoulder blades down your back and together. Hold for five counts. Repeat five times.

To add an extra stretch, gently lift your crossed arms toward your head while continuing to ease your shoulders down your back. Hold for five counts. Repeat five times.

Variation:

This exercise can also be done sitting in an upright position, with arms in front of your chest.

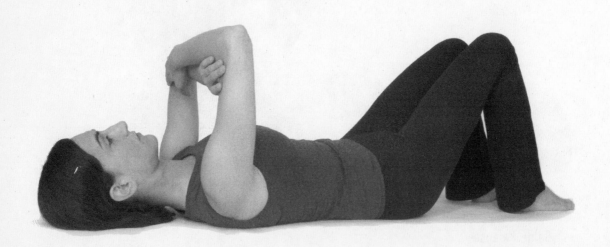

Shoulder Stretch Reclined

Shoulder Rolls

PURPOSE: Relaxation, flexibility in the shoulders, and circulation.

Begin by standing or sitting in an upright position. Engage your abs while keeping the rest of your body relaxed. Roll your shoulders up, then forward and downward, making big circles. Be sure to end each movement with your shoulders back and your chest open. Repeat five times. Reverse the direction by rolling your shoulders backward, then up, then forward again, ending with your chest open and your shoulders back. Repeat five times.

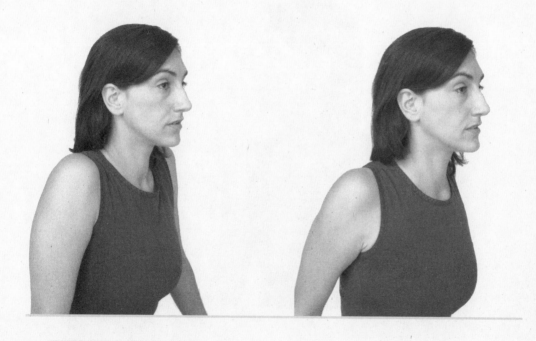

Shoulder Rolls 1 and 2

Neck Turns

PURPOSE: Stretch the neck muscles, promote flexibility of the upper spine, and release neck and upper back tension.

Standing or sitting in an upright position, turn your head and look to one side and hold for five counts. Make sure your shoulders stay down and relaxed. Turn your head back to center, then look to the other side, holding for five counts. Repeat three times each side, alternating sides.

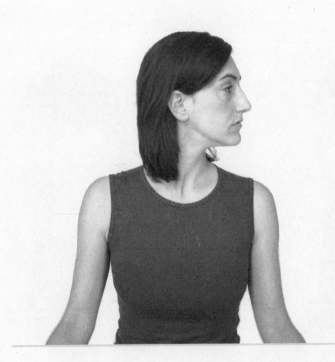

Neck Turns

Neck Circles

PURPOSE: Stretch the neck muscles, promote flexibility of the upper spine, and release neck and upper back tension.

Standing or sitting in an upright position, roll your head by inclining your ear toward your shoulder, then rolling your chin toward your chest, to the other ear, and up. Do not allow your head to rotate to the back, but instead pass through the center with your head erect. Always keep your shoulders down. Repeat two times in each direction.

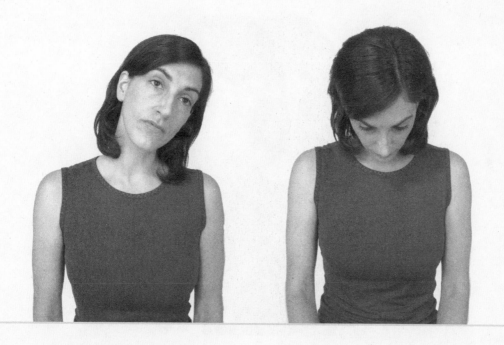

Neck Circles 1 and 2

Shoulder Elevations

PURPOSE: Stretch the shoulders and upper back muscles and release tension in the shoulders and neck.

Standing or sitting in an upright position, engage your abs and lift your shoulders all the way up to your ears. Hold for three counts. Drop your shoulders quickly, as though they are very heavy. Repeat three times.

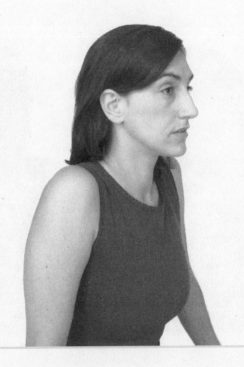

Shoulder Elevations

Neck Exercise

PURPOSE: Strengthen the neck.

Begin in either a standing or a seated position. Keep your neck long, shoulders relaxed, and body upright. Overlap your hands at the back of your neck, right at the base of your head. With your elbows pointing out to the sides, gently press your head into your hands. Hold for ten counts. Repeat three times. Over time, gradually increase the duration of the hold to twenty, and then thirty counts.

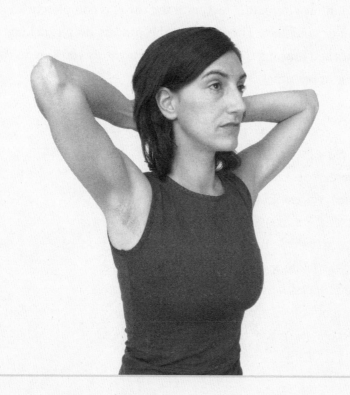

Neck Exercise

Towel Exercise

PURPOSE: Promote circulation in the legs, strengthen and stretch the feet and calves, and help reduce swelling in the feet.

Sit in a chair with your feet touching the ground and your knees bent at a right angle. Place the edge of an unfolded towel under your bare feet, with the length of the towel extending away from you. Starting with one foot, open the toes wide and scrunch them until they grab the towel. Then do the same with the other foot. Continue alternating feet until the towel is completely bunched up under your feet. Then reverse the process by scrunching up your toes and pushing the towel away from you as you extend them. Repeat three times.

Tip: Many of the exercises in this book are done in Pilates stance, which is accomplished by placing your heels together in a "V" position. Your legs should be turned out from the hips so that the back of your thighs are touching. Squeezing your thighs together in this manner helps to engage the buttocks, hips, and outer and inner thighs, which helps stabilize your body. However, if you experience pain, keep your feet in a parallel position.

The Home Stretch

Like the exercises found in the Baby Steps workout, stretching can help decrease muscle tension and promote better posture by reducing stiffness in the joints and muscles. Stretching can also encourage the body to rest and relax, relieving physical as well as emotional stress. Muscle tension can build while performing normal daily activities, such as talking on the phone or carrying your bag to work, so imagine what the stress of new motherhood does to increase muscle tension.

Although the traditional Pilates routine incorporates stretching within many of the exercises, I find it helpful for new moms to do some additional stretching along with their Pilates workout or just by itself. Remember that you are stretching to maintain mobility and flexibility—not to increase your flexibility—so don't push yourself to the point that you strain your muscles. Your joints are still vulnerable to over-stretching and strains due to the lingering effects of the hormone relaxin in your body. You should also guard against straining your muscles when off the mat, like when lifting and toting your baby gear.

Ankle Circles

Lie on your back with your legs raised straight up so that they make a right angle with your body and your feet are stretched up toward the ceiling. If you have lower back pain or are not able to keep your lower back completely on the mat, place either your hands or a folded towel under your tailbone. Begin to rotate your feet in circles, feeling the full range of motion of your ankle joints. Circle ten times in one direction, then reverse.

Ankle Circles

Point/Flex

Lie on your back with your legs raised straight up so that they make a right angle with your body and your feet are stretched up toward the ceiling in Pilates stance. If you have lower back pain or are not able to keep your lower back completely on the mat, place either your hands or a folded towel under your tailbone. Point your toes to the ceiling, then flex them back deeply, pushing your heels to the ceiling. Repeat ten times.

Point/Flex 1

Point/Flex 2

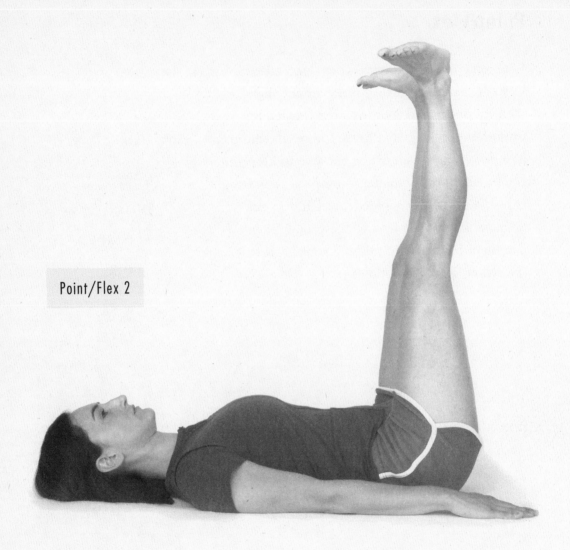

Side Twist

Lie on your back with knees bent and feet together and flat on the floor. Stretch your arms along the floor out to your sides at shoulder height, palms facing up. Let your knees gently fall together over to the right side, turning your head to the left. Make sure that both of your shoulders stay on the ground. Hold for ten counts. Then roll your knees over to the left side and turn your head to the right. Hold for ten counts.

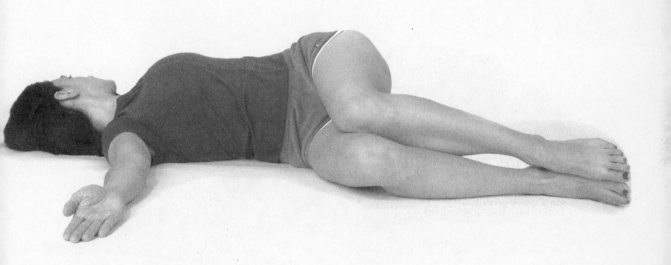

Side Twist

Spine Stretch Release

Position yourself on your hands and knees. Your hands should support your upper body by placing them directly in line with your shoulders. The tops of your feet should rest on the floor. Engage your abdominal muscles and push your body back until you are sitting back on your heels. Stretch your arms forward in front of you with your forearms remaining on the floor. Hold for ten counts. Breathe normally, relaxing your entire body, except your abs, which should be pulling in and up off your thighs to get a maximum stretch in your lower back.

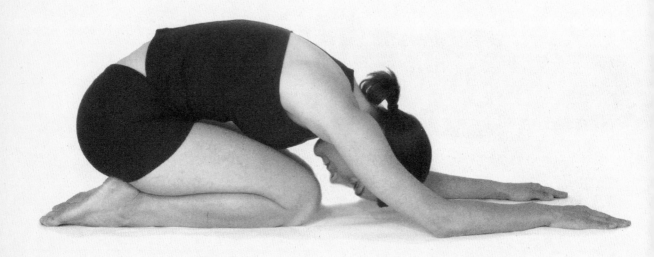

Spine Stretch Release

34

Hip Stretch

Lie on your back with your knees bent in toward your chest. Cross your left ankle over your right knee. Place your left hand on your left knee and right hand under right thigh. Gently push your knee away from your body as you pull your thigh toward you. Hold for ten counts then release. Do the stretch again, then switch to the other leg.

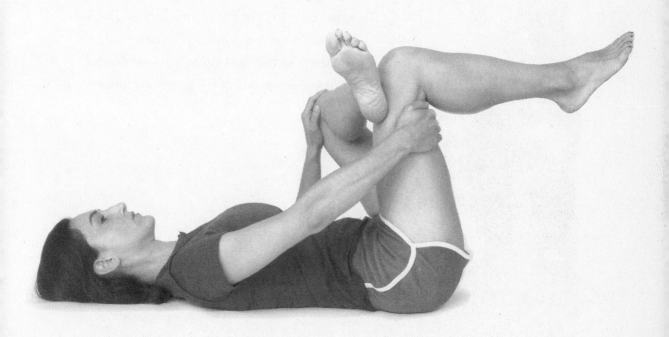

Hip Stretch

Seated Stretch Forward

Sit upright with your legs stretched in front of you and knees soft. Inhale, pull your abs in and gently bend your body forward, walking your hands down your legs as you exhale. Hold on to your calves, ankles, or feet—whichever you can reach comfortably—and continue breathing normally and holding the stretch for three breaths. Each time you exhale, try to take the stretch farther. Do not bounce. Keep your abs in the entire time, and use them to roll back up to a seated position, until you are sitting tall. Repeat two times.

Seated Stretch Forward 1

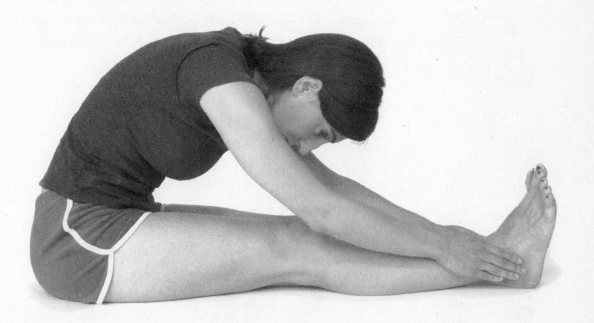

Seated Stretch Forward 2

Kneeling Hip Stretch

Begin in a kneeling position. Raise your left knee and bring your left foot forward, so that your knee is bent at a right angle. Your knee should be in line above your foot—do not let your knee extend beyond your toes. Place both hands on your bent knee to help your balance. Lean into your left leg, lowering your right hip, to stretch forward. Hold for ten counts. Repeat, then switch to the other leg. If you have knee pain, do not do this stretch.

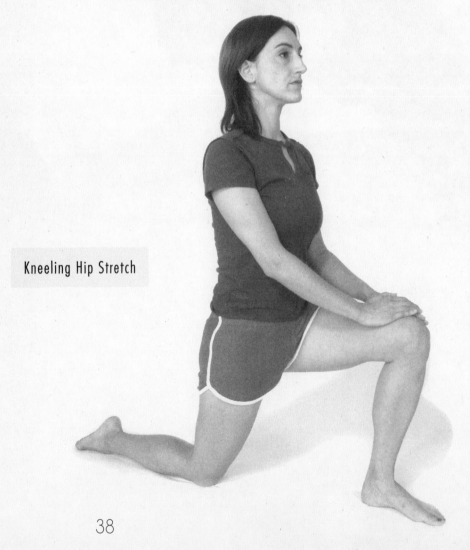

Kneeling Hip Stretch

Chest Stretch

Stand upright with your feet hip-distance apart. Be sure to keep your neck long through this movement and look forward. Clasp your hands behind your back, keeping your palms together. Gently lift your arms up behind you. Only go as high as is comfortable, keeping your shoulders down. This is a gentle stretch. Hold for ten counts. Release. Repeat. If you have shoulder pain, do not do this stretch.

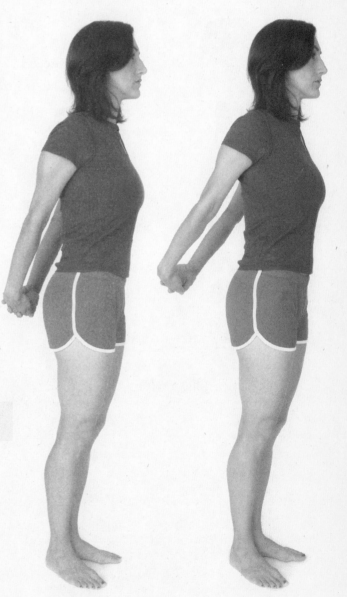

Chest Stretch 1 and 2

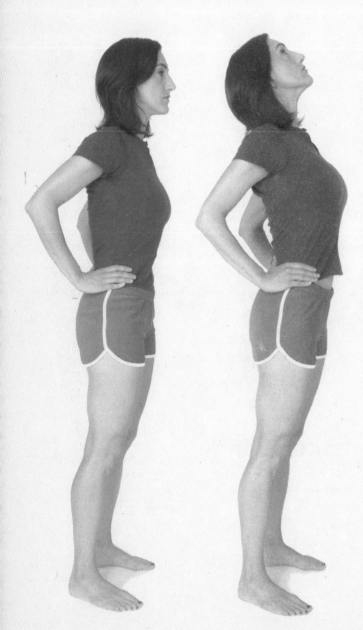

Chest Opener

Stand upright with your feet hip-distance apart and arms bent with hands resting on your hips. Engage your abs, and begin to lift your chest by opening your shoulders wide and squeezing your shoulder blades together in back, bringing your elbows closer together. Allow your head to move naturally with the movement and look slightly upward. Make sure that your neck is lengthening, and do not let your head drop back. Hold for five counts. Repeat. If you have lower back pain, do not do this stretch.

Chest Opener 1 and 2

Wrist Stretches

In a standing or seated position, extend your right arm in front of you at shoulder height. Point your fingers down and your palm away from your body. Grasp your right fingers with your left hand and gently pull the fingers toward you. Keep your palm firm and straight. Hold for ten counts. Do the same on the left hand. Repeat two times. You can also do this exercise with fingers pointing up to the ceiling.

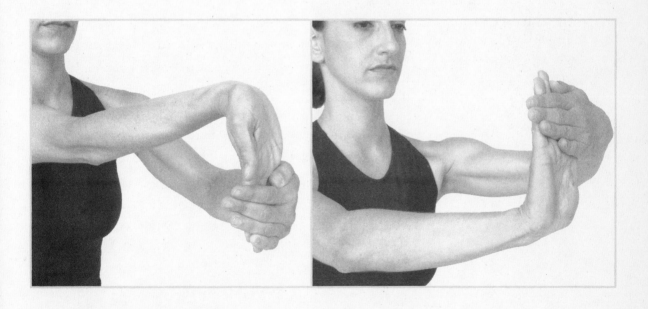

Wrist Stretches 1 and 2

Tip: Recognizing your stress points (the times or situations that cause you stress), and your postural habits during those times, including muscle tension, will allow you to fight against those inclinations naturally. The strength, flexibility, calm, and focus gained through Pilates will improve your posture as well as your ability to deal with stress. You are retraining your body to do what it does naturally—which is take care of itself.

3

The Core Strength Workout

WEEKS 2–6

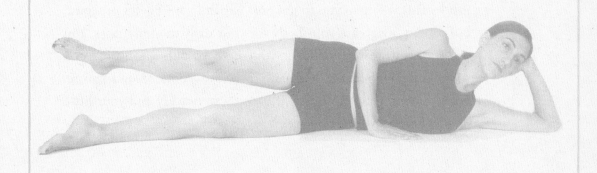

After I overcame my initial fear of taking Ches outside, things were much easier than I expected. I was proud of myself for being able to take this helpless, precious little guy out in the dirty and dangerous world. All I could think about was protecting him from the sun, other people's dirty hands, or the possibility that I could trip and fall. I was overreacting, I know. When I got over those common new-mother fears I felt invincible.

I remember our first walk alone together. I put him in the front carrier and dressed him in the cutest outfit and hat. You know—just in case we saw anyone we knew. We walked to the local video store, returned some movies, and went directly home, which took a total of about twenty minutes. Upon returning home I called my husband at work to tell him about our walk, acting as though I had just accomplished a monumental feat. It is remarkable how something so small can become such a big deal when you are responsible for another life.

Two to six weeks after giving birth, your body still will not feel like your own, so it is important to nurture the healing process with your gentle Pilates routine. By working on pelvic floor and abdominal muscles, you are building a solid base of strength from the inside. This will help you to not only expand your Pilates program, but to also invigorate your body for your daily mommy tasks. You will start getting into a groove with your baby during this time, and soon feeding, changing, and bathing will become second nature. Focus on enjoying this time—it goes by so quickly and your little one will never be this tiny again!

On the outside, one of the first improvements you will notice is better posture, achieved through working on the abdominal muscles and back. These exercises will lengthen your spine, relieve back pain, and will give you the appearance of being taller and slimmer. Don't worry about losing weight quite yet. Eating right to maintain your energy and health is what matters right now. I didn't believe it then, but that soft spare tire around your middle will firm up. Really.

Tip: Walk tall and be proud of your accomplishments—your new baby and your new job as a mother. Not only that, but your waist looks smaller when you stand up straight!

The Core Strength Workout

Begin with the Baby Steps Workout to get your body warmed up, then move on to the Core Strength Workout. If you feel any pain while performing these exercises, stop immediately. Every body recovers at a different pace, so listen to your body and do the movements that feel right for you.

Tummy Tightener

PURPOSE: **Wake up and strengthen the abdominal muscles and strengthen the back.**

Lie on your back with knees bent and feet flat on the floor hip-distance apart. Relax your chest and ribs. Inhale. Pull your abdominal muscles in by imagining you are trying to reach your belly button to your spine, and feel your abs tighten. Hold for five counts. Exhale. Repeat five times.

Do not tense your upper back or push with your feet. Once you have the hang of this, you can do it sitting or standing anywhere you please. Work your way up to holding the movement for ten counts.

Hundred *(modified)*

PURPOSE: **Strengthen the abdominal muscles and increase endurance by focusing on breathing; a warm-up for the exercises that follow.**

Begin by lying on your back. Bend your knees and draw them toward your chest until they are bent at a right angle and your calves are parallel to the ground. Keep your arms down by your sides. Take one deep inhalation through the nose for five counts, then one full exhalation through the mouth for five counts. This is one set. Begin pumping your straight arms up and down, about 4–6 inches off the floor.

Once you have mastered the breathing, lift your head, bringing your chin toward your chest. As you become stronger, extend your legs straight up toward the ceiling. Do ten sets.

Baby Steps/
C-Section
Modification:
If the modified Hundred movement is too difficult or if you have had a C-section, try this further modification: Place your feet on the floor with knees bent, bring your head up, and pump your arms while breathing as stated above. Alternatively, you may keep your knees bent at a right angle with head down (for a tired or tense neck).

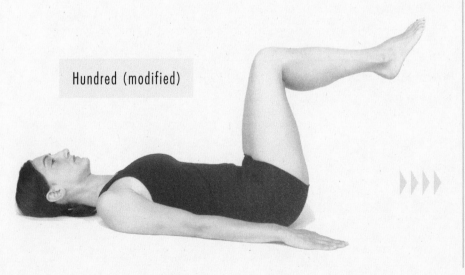

Hundred (modified)

47

Roll Back

PURPOSE: Strengthen the abs and stretch and open the lower back; can be used as a preparation for the Roll Up (page 63).

Sit upright with your knees bent and your feet on the floor hip-distance apart. Lightly hold on to the back of your thighs with your hands. Pull your abdominal muscles in and let your shoulders relax forward. Roll backward by pulling your stomach in so that your tailbone tucks under and tilts forward. Roll down until your waistband touches the mat and hold for five counts. Come back up to a sitting position using only your abdominal muscles, not your arms. As you get stronger, you may roll back farther. Repeat five times.

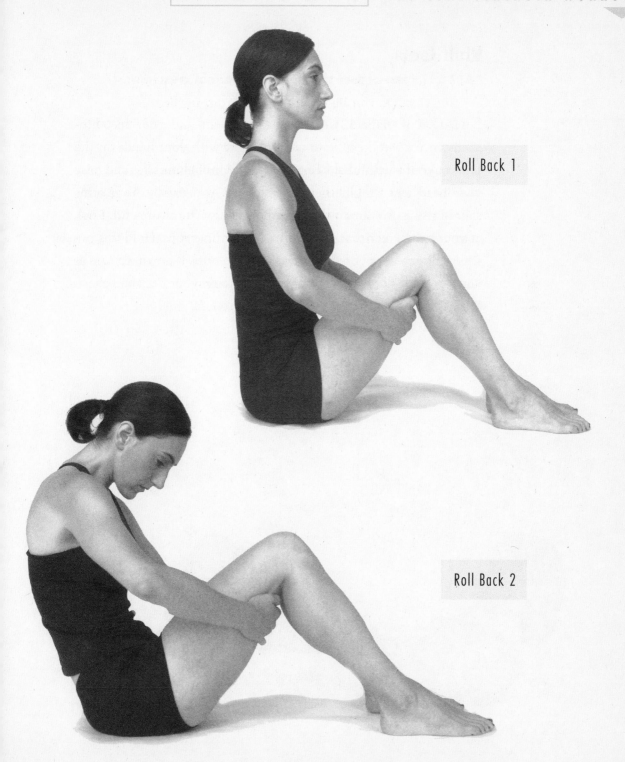

Roll Back 1

Roll Back 2

Half Curl

PURPOSE: **Strengthen the upper abdominal muscles.**

Lying on your back with your knees bent and your feet hip-distance apart, keep your arms straight with your hands on the floor at your sides. Inhale. Engage the abdominal muscles and raise your head and shoulders off the floor as you exhale. Your arms should rise naturally off the ground as you perform the curl. Look at your belly and reach forward with your fingertips. Hold this position for five counts. Inhale as you lower yourself down. Exhale as you reach the floor. Make sure you don't tense your neck and chest. Repeat five times, working your way up to ten.

Half Curl

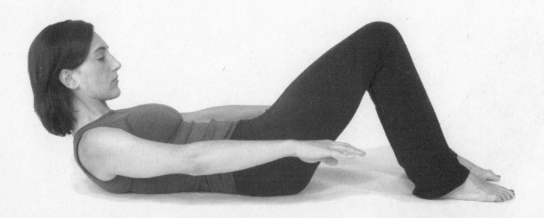

Single Leg Circles *(modified)*

PURPOSE: **Strengthen and stabilize the hips and lengthen and trim the legs.**

Lie on your back with arms relaxed at your sides. Bend your left leg, keeping your foot on the floor, and raise your right leg up to the ceiling. Be sure to keep your head down. Slightly rotate your right leg out from the hip. Make circles by first crossing over your body with your leg, then down, out to the side, and up. Start and stop the circle with your foot over your nose, the center of your body. Keep your leg loose and your hips anchored to the mat with your abdominal muscles. Repeat five times, then reverse the circles five times.

Single Leg Circles (modified)

51

Pelvic Curl

PURPOSE: Release tension in the lower back by lengthening the spine; strengthen the abdominal muscles and pelvic floor.

Lying flat on your back, bend your knees and keep your feet on the ground, hip-distance apart. Completely relax your upper body, reaching your shoulder blades down your back. Engage (or imagine engaging) your lower abdominal muscles by pulling them in. This subtle movement will result in your tailbone reaching away from your body and your spine lengthening.

Hold for ten counts. Release slowly without creating tension in your upper back. Repeat three times in the beginning, working your way up to five, and later ten. Be sure to breathe normally. When you have mastered the Pelvic Curl, add a Kegel (page 18) while you hold the curl. Release the Kegel hold as you release the curl position.

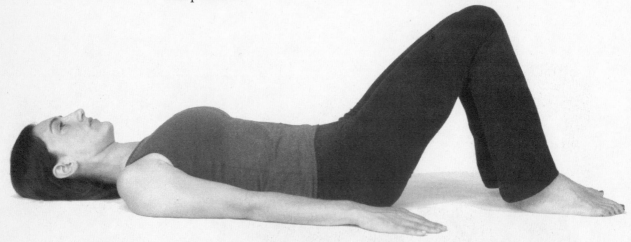

Pelvic Curl

52

Single Leg Stretch *(modified)*

PURPOSE: **Strengthen the abs and stretch the back of the legs.**

Lying on your back, bend your right knee to your chest. Place your right hand on the right ankle and left hand on right knee. Bring your head up and chin to your chest and lift your left leg at a 45-degree angle to the ground. If you have knee pain, place your hands under your knees when drawing your leg toward your body. Remember that this is not just an abdominal exercise but also a stretch for the back of your legs (hamstrings), so be sure to feel the stretch in your right leg.

Switch legs, pulling your left knee in to your chest, with your left hand on the left ankle and right hand on left knee. Keep your legs in alignment when bent or straight by directing them down the centerline of your body. Repeat ten times and do five sets.

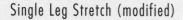

Single Leg Stretch (modified)

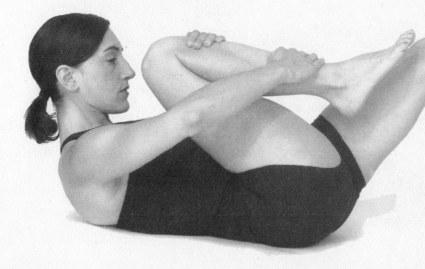

Double Leg Stretch *(modified)*

PURPOSE: Strengthen the abs and stretch the body.

Lying on your back, bring both knees into your chest, holding on to your ankles. If you have knee pain, place your hands under your knees. Bring your head up and chin toward your chest. Inhale. Raise your arms over your head so they are straight and close to your ears. At the same time extend your legs straight at a 45-degree angle to the ground. If you have back pain, modify by raising your legs higher.

Circle your arms out to the sides and exhale. Complete the arm circle by reaching for your ankles as you pull your knees back in to your chest. Your legs should stay together throughout the exercise. Repeat five to ten times.

Double Leg Stretch 1

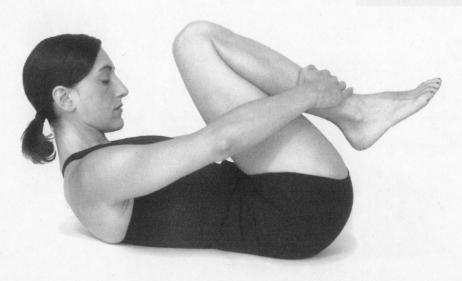

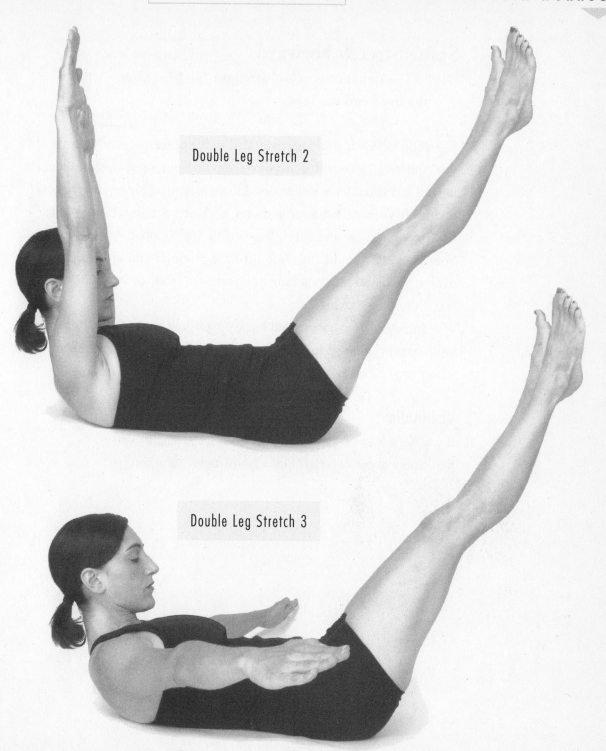

Double Leg Stretch 2

Double Leg Stretch 3

Spine Stretch Forward

PURPOSE: Enhance postural strength (abs, back) and stretch the back and the legs.

Sit up tall with your legs extended to the outer edges of the mat and feet flexed. Reach your arms in front of you, shoulder height and shoulder-width apart. Inhale as you squeeze your buttocks, lift your pelvic floor muscles, and sit up taller. Bring your chin to your chest and reach forward by rolling down your spine. Your stomach should continue lifting, as though you are bending over a big ball. Keep reaching your arms in front of you with relaxed shoulders. Exhale.

Inhale as you start to roll back up, pulling your abs in. Reach your fingers forward as you continue to sit up tall. Keep lifting when you reach the top, then exhale. Repeat three to five times.

Modification:

If you have back or knee pain, bend your knees slightly, or sit on a firm pillow to position your hips slightly higher than your feet.

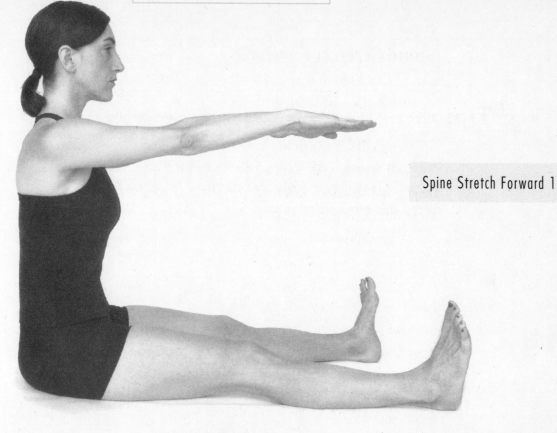

Spine Stretch Forward 1

Spine Stretch Forward 2

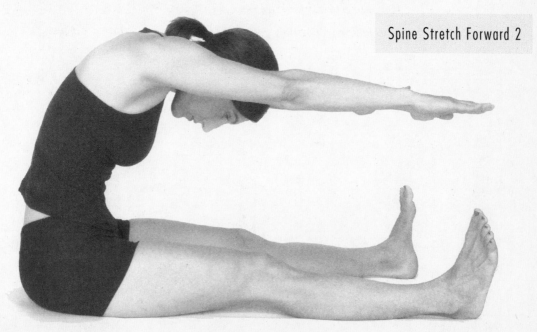

▶▶▶▶ **Tip:** Remember to breathe, while performing the exercises and always. Sometimes we forget to breathe when we are concentrating on the exercises or when we lose patience or talk too much! Breathing encourages circulation, helps you think clearly, and promotes relaxation.

4

Getting Your Body
Back Workout

AFTER 6 WEEKS

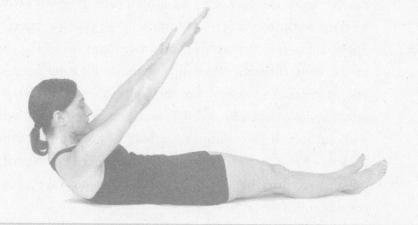

Your six weeks postpartum doctor's appointment is a milestone of sorts. Your OB/GYN will likely approve more physical activity and tell you it is okay to resume sexual activity. This is both scary and exciting—you can no longer rely upon your postpartum haze as an excuse to be a blob. But on the other hand, you are human again, more or less. Sure, you are still occasionally allowed to be sleepy, grumpy, bashful, or dopey, but it's time to step up and get with the program.

If you have been following the program in this book regularly, six weeks after the birth of your baby, your abdominal muscles will feel alive, your lower back will be in shape, and your whole body will have become stronger. You will also have learned to work your abdominal muscles by pulling in, not pushing out. By doing this, you have started to engage the deepest muscles of your core (the transverse abdominis muscles), which support your torso like an internal corset. Your doctor will also be impressed with your promising pelvic floor control. This is a good time to ask him or her questions about your workout plans, weight loss, and nutrition.

If after six weeks, you or your doctor has decided that you are not yet up to the task of trying more challenging workouts, keep working on the basics. It is great to challenge yourself, but it is more important to feel comfortable and ready to move on. The exercises in the Core Strength Workout are the foundation for regaining your strength. The exercises in the Getting Your Body Back Workout that follow build on this foundation. Start slowly with this workout so that you continue to move forward instead of moving back due to injury or fatigue. Also, if you experience vaginal bleeding, you are probably doing too much too soon. Take a break and consult your doctor.

Getting Your Body Back Workout

How your body recovers from pregnancy and labor are very specific to you as an individual. When you can do the Core Strength Workout without modifications, or with minimal modifications, move on to the Getting Your Body Back Workout. Six weeks postpartum is the standard green light to step up your physical activity level. If it takes longer, or you find yourself recovering more quickly, make adjustments to your workout as you see fit. Do the Core Strength Workout routine four times per week for at least three weeks before moving on to the more challenging routines that follow.

Hundred

PURPOSE: **Strengthen the abdominal muscles
and increase endurance by focusing on
breathing; a warm-up for the exercises
that follow.**

Begin by lying on your back. Raise your legs
straight up toward the ceiling so that your body
and legs form a 90-degree angle. Keep your arms down
by your sides. Take one deep inhalation through the
nose for five counts, then one full exhalation through
the mouth for five counts. This is one set. Begin
pumping your straight arms up and down, about 4–6
inches off the floor. Once you have mastered the
breathing, lift your head and bring your chin toward
your chest. As you become stronger, lower your legs
toward the ground. Do ten sets.

Modification:

*If you have lower back pain, keep your legs slightly
bent or bent at a right angle.*

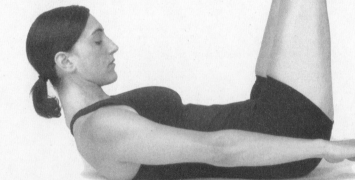

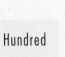

Hundred

Roll Up

PURPOSE: **Strengthen the abs and stretch the spine and back of the legs.**

Lie on your back with your legs slightly bent and feet in Pilates stance, heels on the mat. Extend your arms straight overhead so that they are parallel to your ears, shoulder-width apart. Raise your head and inhale, then lift your arms toward the ceiling and begin rolling up, pulling your abdominal muscles in while reaching arms forward. Exhale as you reach beyond your toes.

Inhale, pull your abs in, and begin to roll back down, trying to touch each vertebra consecutively on the mat until you are lying flat again with arms up by your ears. Exhale as you return to the starting position. If you cannot roll up smoothly, keep your arms at your sides during the roll up and down. Repeat three to five times.

Modification:
Bend your knees slightly and keep your arms by your sides if you cannot roll up smoothly.

C-Section Modification:
Refer to the Roll Back (page 66) until you are well on your way to being healed.

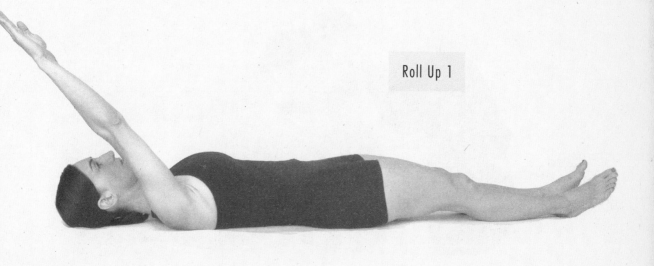

Roll Up 1

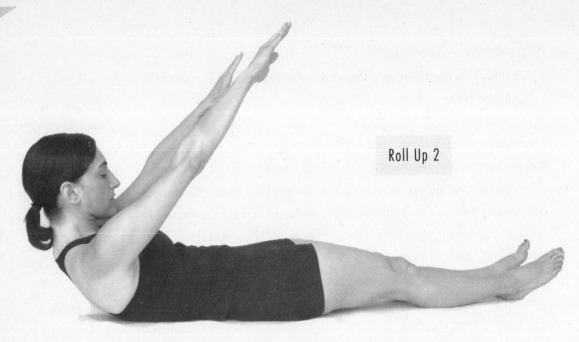

Roll Up 2

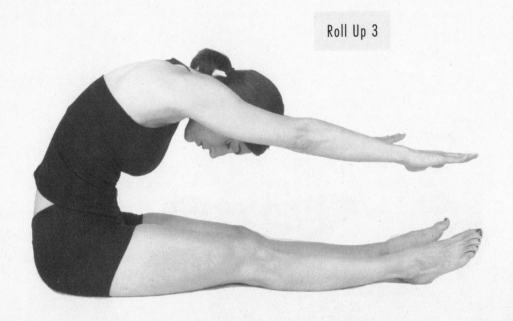

Roll Up 3

Single Leg Circles

PURPOSE: **Strengthen and stabilize the hips and lengthen and trim the legs.**

Lie on your back with arms relaxed at your sides. Keeping your left leg straight, raise your right leg up to the ceiling. Be sure to keep your head down. Slightly rotate your right leg out from the hip. Make circles by first crossing over your body with your leg, then down, out to the side, and up. Start and stop the circle with your foot over your nose, the center of your body. Keep your leg loose and your hips anchored to the mat with your abdominal muscles. Repeat five times, then reverse the circles five times.

Modification/ C-Section Modification:

If you cannot keep your back flat or you feel a strain in your knee, start by doing this exercise with one leg bent, foot on the floor, while making circles with the other leg.

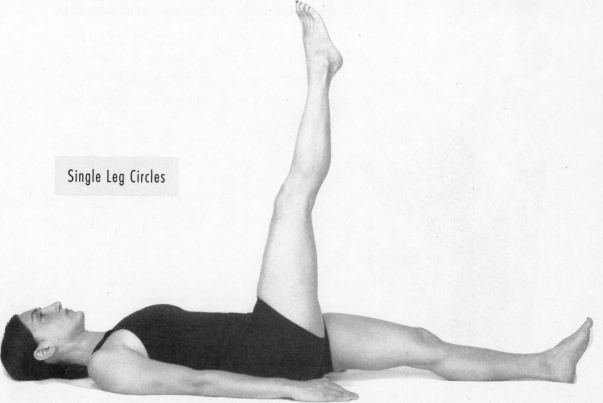

Single Leg Circles

Roll Back

PURPOSE: Strengthen the abs, stretch and open the lower back; can be used as a preparation for the Roll Up (page 63) and Rolling Like a Ball (page 156).

Sit upright with your knees bent and your feet on the floor hip-distance apart. Lightly hold on to the back of your thighs with your hands. Pull your abdominal muscles in and let your shoulders relax forward. Roll backward by pulling your stomach in so that your tailbone tucks under and tilts forward. Roll down until your waistband touches the mat and hold for five counts. Come back up to a sitting position using only your abdominal muscles, not your arms. As you get stronger, you may roll back farther. Repeat five times.

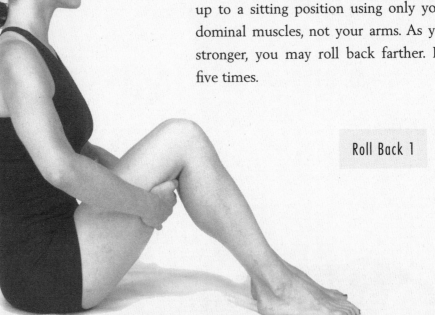

Roll Back 1

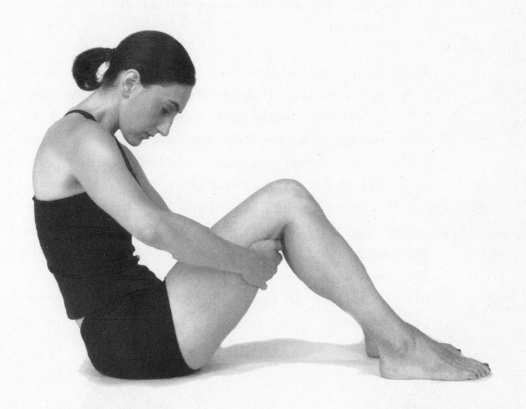

Roll Back 2

Pelvic Curl

PURPOSE: Release tension in the lower back by lengthening the spine; strengthen the abdominal muscles and pelvic floor.

Lying flat on your back, bend your knees and keep your feet on the ground, hip-distance apart. Completely relax your upper body, reaching your shoulder blades down your back. Engage (or imagine engaging) your lower abdominal muscles by pulling them in. This subtle movement will result in your tailbone reaching away from your body and your spine lengthening.

Hold for ten counts. Release slowly without creating tension in your upper back. Repeat three times in the beginning, working your way up to five, and later ten. Make sure you breathe normally. When you have mastered the Pelvic Curl, add a Kegel (page 18) while you hold the curl. Release the Kegel hold as you release the curl position.

Pelvic Curl

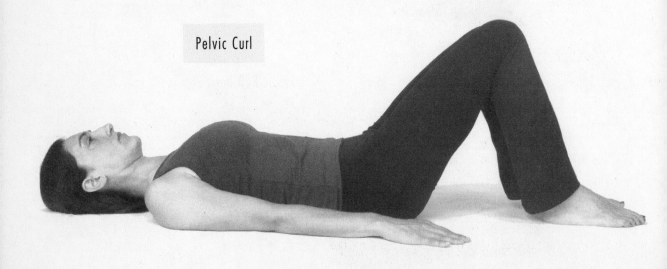

Single Leg Stretch

PURPOSE: **Strengthen the abs and stretch the back of the legs.**

Lying on your back, bend your right knee to your chest. Place your right hand on the right ankle and left hand on right knee. Bring your head up and chin to your chest and lift your left leg at a 45-degree angle to the ground. Remember that this is not just an abdominal exercise but also a stretch for the back of your legs (hamstrings), so be sure to feel the stretch in your right leg.

Switch legs, pulling your left knee into your chest, with your left hand on the left ankle and right hand on left knee. Keep your legs in alignment when bent or straight by directing them down the centerline of your body. Repeat ten times and do five sets. As you become stronger, you may lower your legs toward the floor.

Modification:
If you have knee pain, place your hands under your knees. If you have lower back pain, keep your legs higher with your heels over your hips.

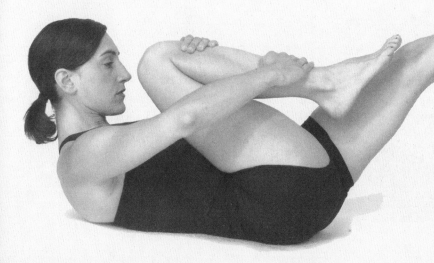

Single Leg Stretch

Double Leg Stretch

PURPOSE: Strengthen the abs and stretch the body.

Lying on your back, bring both knees into your chest, holding on to your ankles. Bring your head up and chin toward your chest. Inhale. Raise your arms over your head so they are straight and close to your ears. At the same time, extend your legs straight at a 45-degree angle to the ground.

Circle your arms out to the sides and exhale. Complete the arm circle by reaching for your ankles as you pull your knees back in to your chest. Your legs should stay together throughout the exercise. Repeat five to ten times. As you become stronger, you may lower your legs toward the floor.

Modification:

If you have knee pain, place your hands under your knees. If you have back pain, raise your legs higher off the mat.

Double Leg Stretch 1

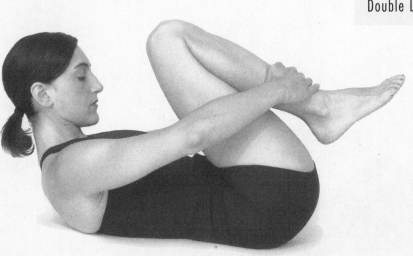

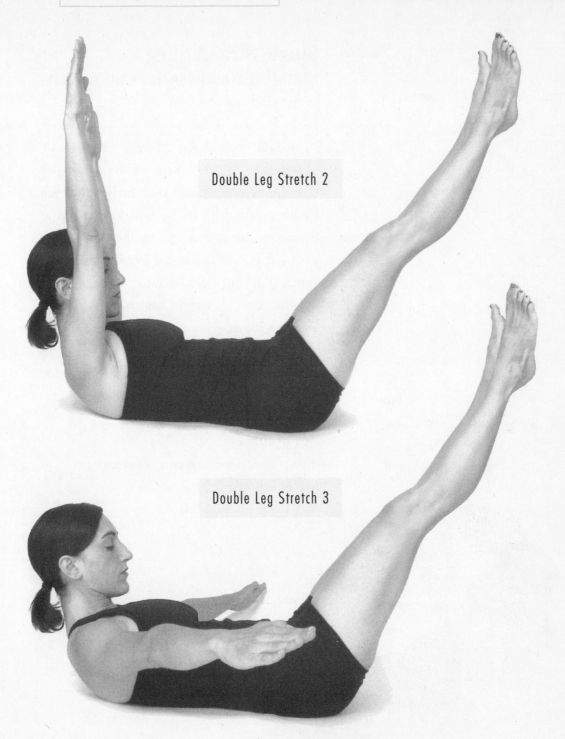

Double Leg Stretch 2

Double Leg Stretch 3

71

Single Straight Leg

PURPOSE: **Stretch the legs while strengthening the abs.**

Lying on your back, bring your head up and chin to chest. Keeping your right leg straight, raise it toward your body and reach for your right calf with both hands. Keep your shoulders pressed down to the mat. Raise your left leg off the mat a few inches as you gently pull your right leg into your body, feeling the stretch in your hamstring. Alternate legs by scissoring them through the air and pull your left leg into your body. Repeat ten times and do five sets. As you become stronger, you may lower your legs toward the floor.

Modification:

If you have lower back pain, keep your extended leg higher off the mat.

Single Straight Leg

Crisscross *(modified)*

PURPOSE: Strengthen the oblique muscles and trim the waistline.

Lie on your back with knees bent and feet flat on the mat hip-distance apart. Extend your arms in front of you with one hand on top of the other. Bring your head up, chin to chest. Use your obliques (side ab muscles) to lift your upper body slightly by pressing your ribs down and rolling your shoulders off the mat. Reach your hands to the right of your knees and hold for one count. Then twist and reach to the left of your knees. Try not to rest between sides. Stabilize your body with your abs; only your upper body should twist. Do three sets.

Crisscross (modified)

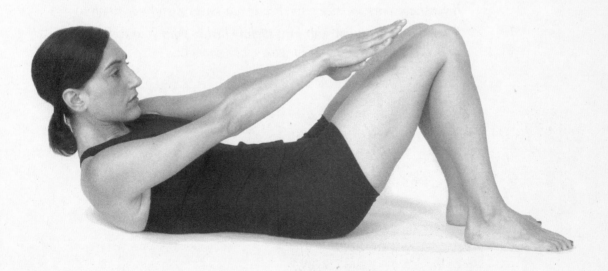

Spine Stretch Forward

PURPOSE: Enhance postural strength (abs, back) and stretch the back and the legs.

Sit up tall with your legs extended to the outer edges of the mat and feet flexed. Reach your arms in front of you, shoulder height and shoulder-width apart. Inhale as you squeeze your buttocks, lift your pelvic floor muscles, and sit up taller. Bring your chin to your chest and reach forward by rolling down your spine. Your stomach should continue lifting, as though you are bending over a big ball. Keep reaching your arms in front of you with relaxed shoulders. Exhale.

Inhale as you start to roll back up, pulling your abs in. Reach your fingers forward as you continue to sit up tall. Keep lifting when you reach the top, then exhale. Repeat three to five times.

Modification:

If you have back or knee pain, bend your knees slightly, or sit on a firm pillow to position your hips slightly higher than your feet.

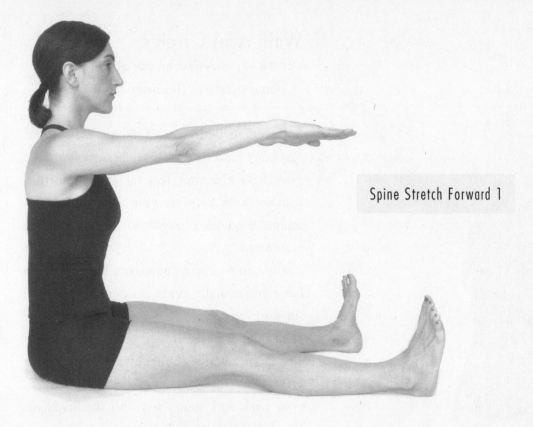

Spine Stretch Forward 1

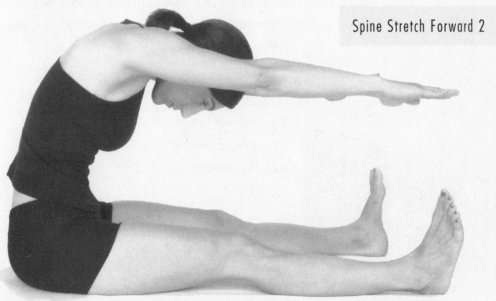

Spine Stretch Forward 2

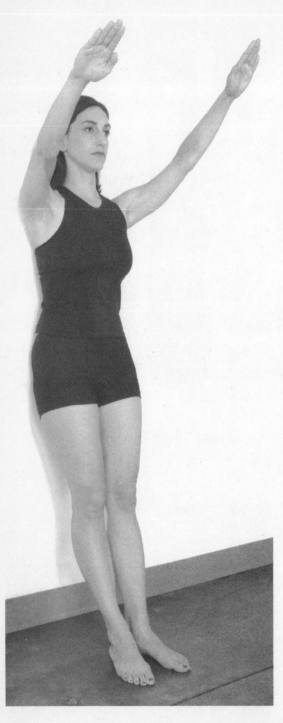

Wall: Arm Circles

PURPOSE: Strengthen the abs and back and increase shoulder mobility.

Standing with feet in Pilates stance and your back against a wall, step your feet away from the wall, just far enough so that you are able to press your entire back flat against the wall. Engage your abs to stabilize your torso.

Begin to circle your arms, keeping them loose and straight. Bring your arms out to the sides, up over the shoulders, and then down in front of your chest. Inhale as your arms go up and exhale as they come down. Remember to keep your shoulder blades reaching down your back and your chest and shoulders relaxed. Your arms should stay in your peripheral vision. Repeat three to five times, then reverse the circles.

Variation:
You may use two- to three-pound weights with this exercise.

Wall: Arm Circles

Wall: Rolling Down

PURPOSE: Strengthen the abs, stretch the back, and promote relaxation.

Standing with your back against a wall, bring your chin to your chest. Relax your shoulders and place your arms at your sides. Keeping your stomach lifted and pressed in to your spine, start to peel your back off the wall beginning with the shoulders, removing one vertebra at a time. Roll down to your waist while pressing your lower back against the wall by keeping your abs pulled in tight. Your fingers will likely be at knee level.

Maintain stillness in your body, feeling gravity pull you down. Let your arms hang heavy and make a few tiny, loose, effortless circles in one direction. Then reverse the direction of the circles. Try to let your arms stop moving on their own.

Pull your abs in and up, slowly rolling back up the wall, pressing each vertebra individually into the wall until you are standing erect.

Wall: Rolling Down 1

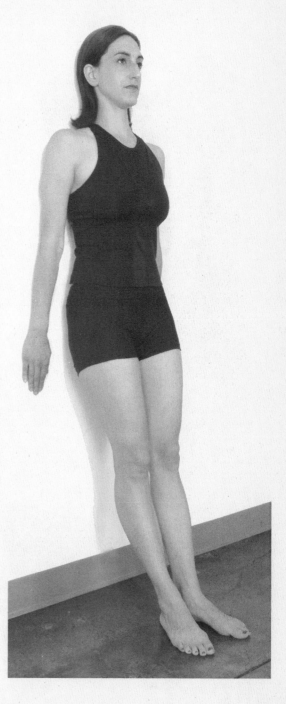

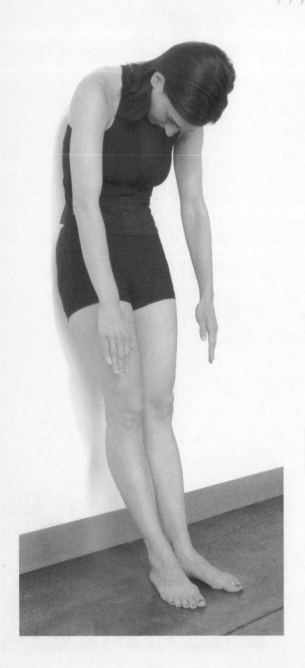

Tip: Set goals for yourself but keep them realistic. They should not stress you out, only inspire you. Remember that your objective is to have a healthier, stronger, and therefore more fabulous body, so don't focus on the scale. You are creating your own version of perfection. These workouts will redistribute the weight, reshape the body, and help you lose inches.

Wall: Rolling Down 2

5

Target Your Trouble Zones:

Abs, Butt, Legs, Arms

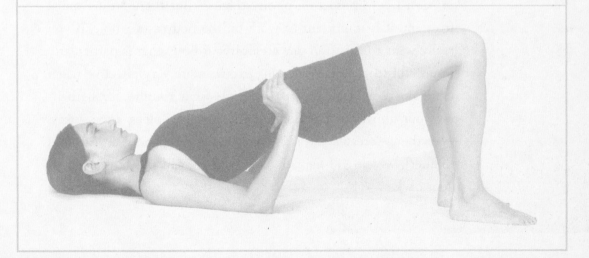

Months one through three were downright blissful. It was August through October and the weather was beautiful. Every day just before lunch we would gather our things and head out. For short walks I packed minimally because I had him in the front carrier and didn't want to load myself down. This meant that I carried Ches, a burp cloth, his hat, and some cash. No diapers? Sounds risky, I know, but I didn't venture far from home. We would walk around the neighborhood, buy lunch, perhaps sit in the park, and then go home. What was great about wearing Ches on my chest was that I had free hands, and I loved the feeling of having him so close to me. He mostly slept but I like to think we both enjoyed those walks.

Let's face it, no matter how much you exercised or how kind nature (genetics) has been to you, pregnancy changed your body and how you see yourself. Positive self-image is always important, but especially now, when you are constantly fatigued and feeling less than perfect. I frequently hear women say, "I hate my arms," or "Can I get liposuction on my thighs?" But there are no quick fixes and it is important to work on the body as a whole. If you really want to focus on one area of your body that is particularly distasteful to you, the following exercises are very effective when done alone or when incorporated into your routine. Strengthening your upper body, abdominal muscles, back, legs, arms—okay, everything—creates the illusion of being long and graceful (and thinner), which will happen soon enough, and prevents stress to your back.

Tip: Make sure you have mastered the first few workouts in this book before jumping into the exercises that follow.

The Abs

Okay, so you don't even want to look at your stomach right now. But getting your abdominal muscles back into shape is the aim of post-pregnancy Pilates workouts. Think of the abdominal muscles as the control center of your body, dictating your overall strength, quality of your posture, and the focus of your next trip to the beach. Follow these exercises to strengthen and flatten your abs in no time.

Hundred

PURPOSE: Strengthen the abdominal muscles and increase endurance by focusing on breathing; a warm-up for the exercises that follow.

Begin by lying on your back. Raise your legs straight up toward the ceiling so that your body and legs form a 90-degree angle. Keep your arms down by your sides. Take one deep inhalation through the nose for five counts, then one full exhalation through the mouth for five counts. This is one set. Begin pumping your straight arms up and down, about 4–6 inches off the floor. Once you have mastered the breathing, lift your head and bring your chin toward your chest. As you become stronger, lower your legs toward the ground. Do ten sets.

Baby Steps/C-Section Modification:

Place your feet on the floor with knees bent, bring your head up and pump your arms while breathing as stated above. Alternatively, you may keep your knees bent at a right angle with head down (for a tired or tense neck) or up.

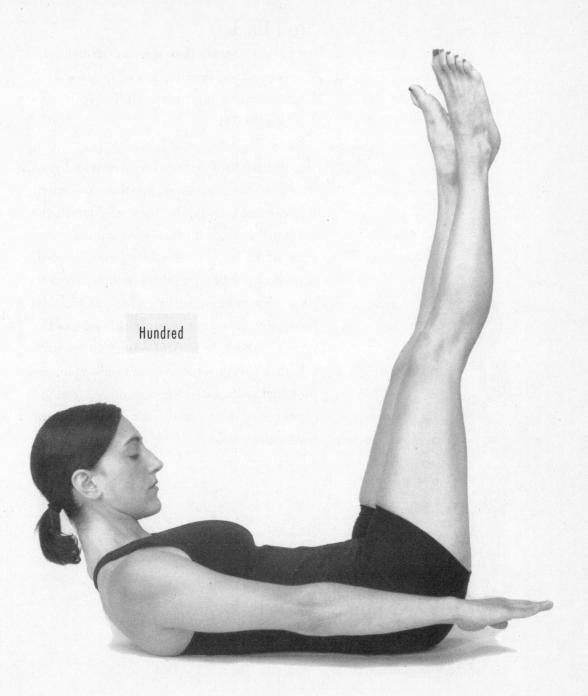

Hundred

Roll Back

PURPOSE: Strengthen the abs, stretch and open the lower back; can be used as a preparation for the Roll Up (page 63).

Sit upright with your knees bent and your feet on the floor hip-distance apart. Lightly hold on to the back of your thighs with your hands. Pull your abdominal muscles in and let your shoulders relax forward. Roll backward by pulling your stomach in so that your tailbone tucks under and tilts forward. Roll down until your waistband touches the mat and hold for five counts. Come back up to a sitting position using only your abdominal muscles, not your arms. As you get stronger, you may roll back farther. Repeat five times.

Roll Back 1

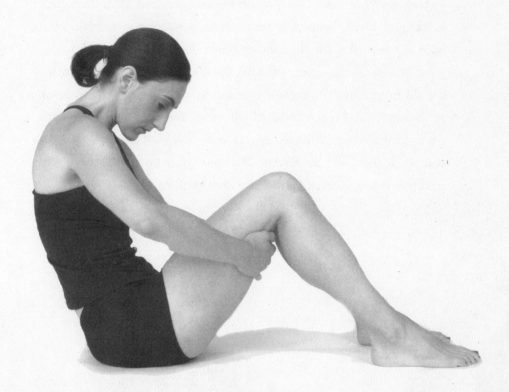

Roll Back 2

Half Curl

PURPOSE: Strengthen the upper abdominal muscles.

Lying on your back with your knees bent and your feet hip-distance apart, keep your arms straight with your hands on the floor at your sides. Inhale. Engage the abdominal muscles and raise your head and shoulders off the floor as you exhale. Your arms should rise naturally off the ground as you perform the curl. Look at your belly and reach forward with your fingertips. Hold this position for five counts. Inhale as you lower yourself down. Exhale as you reach the floor. Be sure not to tense your neck and chest. Repeat five times, working your way up to ten.

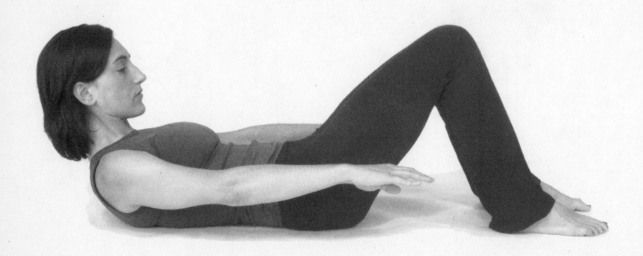

Half Curl

Single Leg Stretch

PURPOSE: Strengthen the abs and stretch the back of the legs.

Lying on your back, bend your right knee to your chest. Place your right hand on the right ankle and left hand on right knee. Bring your head up and chin to your chest and lift your left leg at a 45-degree angle to the ground. Remember that this is not just an abdominal exercise but also a stretch for the back of your legs (hamstrings), so be sure to feel the stretch in your right leg.

Switch legs, pulling your left knee into your chest, with your left hand on the left ankle and right hand on left knee. Keep your legs in alignment when bent or straight by directing them down the centerline of your body. Repeat ten times and do five sets.

Modification:

If you have knee pain, place your hands under your knees. If you have lower back pain, keep your legs higher, with your heels over your legs.

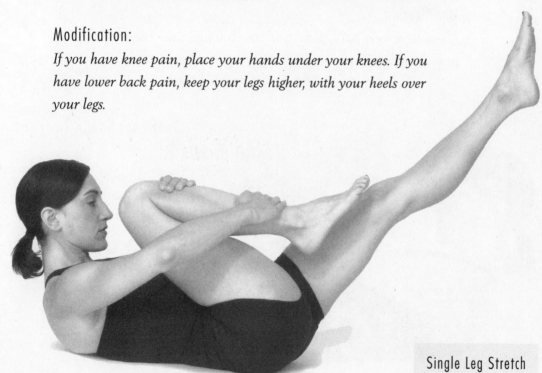

Single Leg Stretch

87

Double Leg Stretch

PURPOSE: **Strengthen the abs and stretch the body.**

Lying on your back, bring both knees in to your chest, holding on to your ankles. Bring your head up and chin toward your chest. Inhale. Raise your arms over your head so they are straight and close to your ears. At the same time, extend your legs straight at a 45-degree angle to the ground.

Circle your arms out to the sides and exhale. Complete the arm circle by reaching for your ankles as you pull your knees back into your chest. Your legs should stay together throughout the exercise. Repeat five to ten times.

Modification:

If you have knee pain, place your hands under your knees. If you have back pain, raise your legs higher off the mat.

Double Leg Stretch 1

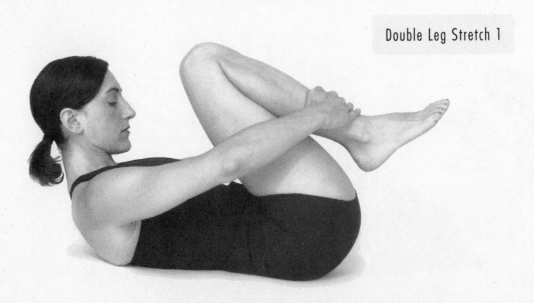

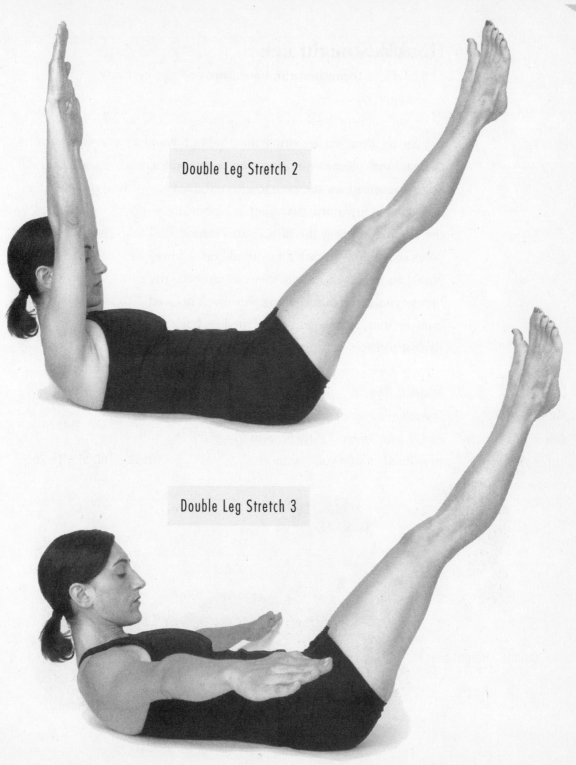

Double Leg Stretch 2

Double Leg Stretch 3

Double Straight Leg

PURPOSE: Strengthen the lower and upper abs.

Lying on your back with hands behind your head and elbows pointing out to the sides, bring your head up and chin to chest. Raise your legs straight up until your feet are pointing to the ceiling, keeping them in Pilates stance. Pull your abdominal muscles in, inhale, and lower your legs together. Lower them as close to the mat as you can while keeping your back pressed into the mat. Exhale and bring the legs back up. Repeat five to ten times.

C-Section Modification:
Leave this exercise out until you are completely healed.

Modification:
If you have lower back pain, keep your legs higher with knees slightly bent and/or place your hands under your buttocks.

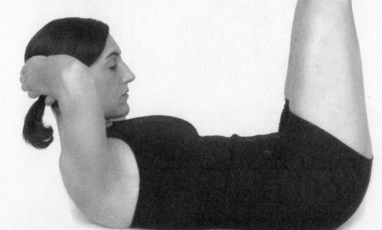

Double Straight Leg 1

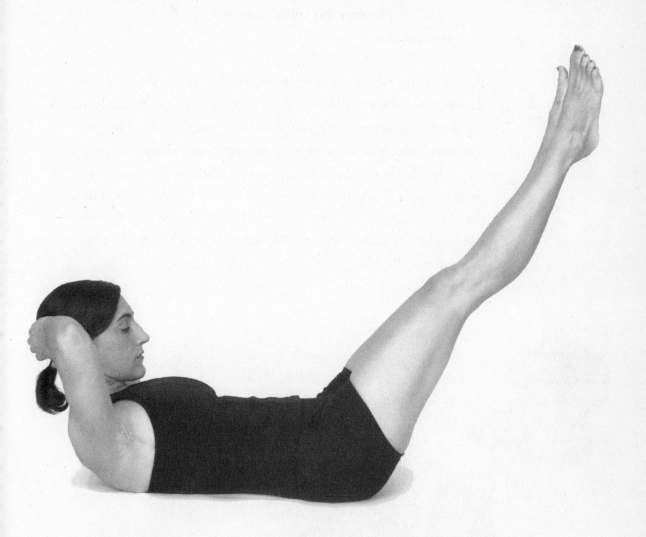

Double Straight Leg 2

Crisscross *(modified)*

PURPOSE: **Strengthen the oblique muscles and trim the waistline.**

Lie on your back with knees bent and feet flat on the mat hip-distance apart. Extend your arms in front of you with one hand on top of the other. Bring your head up, chin to chest. Use your obliques (side ab muscles) to lift your upper body slightly by pressing your ribs down and rolling your shoulders off the mat. Reach your hands to the right of your knees and hold for one count. Then twist and reach to the left of your knees. Try not to rest between sides. Stabilize with your abs; only your upper body should twist. Do three sets.

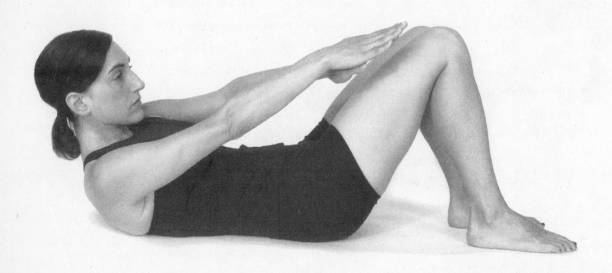

Crisscross (modified)

Butt

The true magic of postpartum Pilates, for me, manifested itself in the waist, hip, and buttocks area. I whittled down my waist, ridding myself of that horrifying hip "shelf" that had installed itself just above my buttocks during pregnancy. By doing the following exercises, you will lift your butt and smooth out the hip area.

Side Kicks: Front/Back *(Intermediate)*
PURPOSE: **Lengthen and tone the legs, hips, and buttocks.**

Lie on your side, lining up your back with the edge of your mat. Rest your head on your hand, with the other hand on the mat in front of your stomach. Bring your legs in front of you at a 45-degree angle (home position). Engage your abdominal muscles to stabilize the upper body, with the hips stacked on top of each other throughout the exercise. Keep your leg movements flowing and smooth.

With both legs straight, lift the top leg to hip height. Slightly rotate the leg out from the hip (with knee turned toward the ceiling), keeping your leg hip height throughout the exercise. Engage your abdominal muscles and kick your leg to the front with energy. Stretch the leg long on the back kick. Repeat five to ten times, then do a set of Side Kicks: Beats with Knee Lifts (page 95), then repeat on the other side.

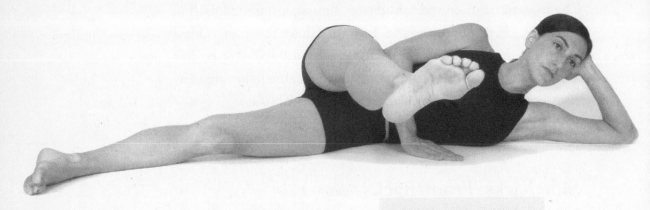

Side Kicks: Front/Back 1

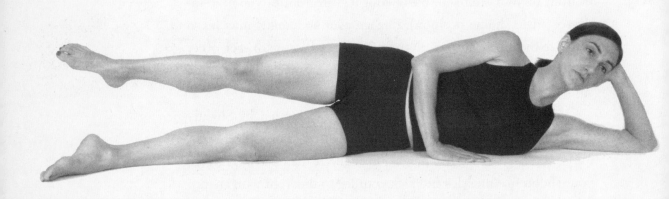

Side Kicks: Front/Back 2

Side Kick: Beats with Knee Lifts

PURPOSE: Strengthen the lower back, inner and outer thighs, and butt.

Lie on your stomach with your forehead resting on the back of your hands and your elbows pointing out to the sides. Relax your shoulders and lift your belly off the mat to support your lower back. With your legs straight and feet in Pilates stance, lift your legs (and knees) off the mat and beat your inner thighs together. Repeat three sets of ten repetitions. Then, turn to your other side and repeat Side Kicks: Front/Back.

Variation:

Relaxing your upper body, bend your knees and lift them off the mat, and bring your heels toward your buttocks. This is a great exercise to "lift" your butt. Hold for five counts, then release. Repeat three times.

Transitional Leg Beats

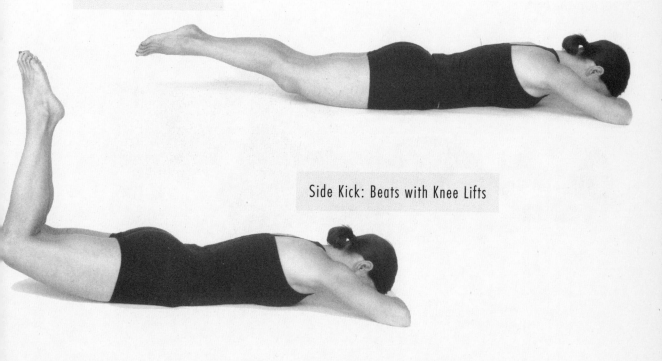

Side Kick: Beats with Knee Lifts

Shoulder Bridge

PURPOSE: Strengthen the abs and legs and lift the buttocks.

Lie on your back with knees bent, legs hip-distance apart, and feet flat on the floor. Lift your hips off the mat until your body makes a straight plane. Support your hips with your hands, keeping your elbows and upper arms on the mat. Inhale. Straighten your right leg, pointing your toes to the ceiling. Flex your foot as you bring it back to knee level. Keep your hips even by tightening your abdominal muscles. Exhale. Repeat three times, then switch legs.

Variation:
Do this exercise with your arms at your sides, relying on your abs to support the body.

Modification:
If you find this exercise too challenging, do the Pelvic Curl (page 20) until you are ready for the Shoulder Bridge.

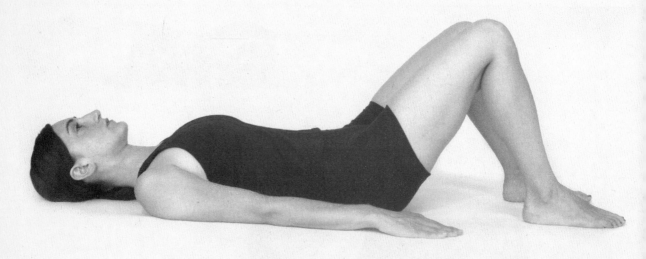

Shoulder Bridge 1

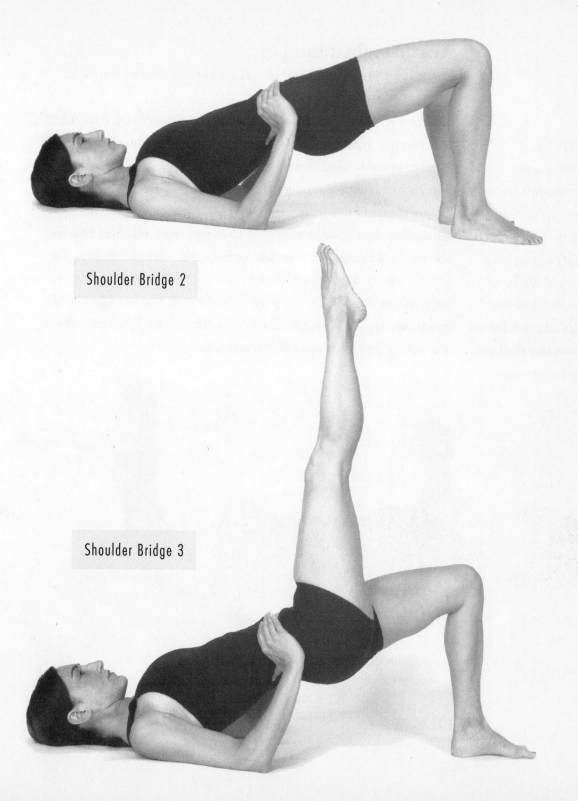

Shoulder Bridge 2

Shoulder Bridge 3

Arm Weights: Lunges

PURPOSE: Strengthen the abs, legs, butt, and arms.

Variation:

Holding arm weights, raise your arms in front of you to shoulder height as you lunge forward. Pull your arms back to your sides as you return to a standing position.

Stand with your feet hip-distance apart and arms by your sides, keeping your neck long and your gaze straight ahead. With weights in each hand, keep your arms down at your sides. Take a step forward with your right leg and bend your left knee. Make sure your right knee does not go past your toes and that your torso remains upright (not leaning over your leg). Your left heel will rise off the floor slightly as your left knee bends toward the floor. Engage your abdominal muscles and push yourself back up to a standing position. Repeat by stepping forward with the left leg. Do ten repetitions on each leg, alternating legs, for one set. Work up to two sets, taking a short break in between.

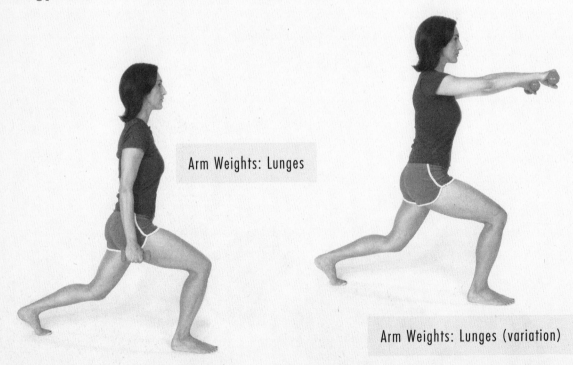

Arm Weights: Lunges

Arm Weights: Lunges (variation)

Wall: Squat

PURPOSE: Strengthen the buttocks, legs, abs, and back.

Stand with your back against a wall and your feet hip-distance apart. Move your feet away from the wall so that when you squat, your knees will not extend over your toes. Lift your abs and begin to slide down the wall into a sitting position until your thighs are parallel to the floor and your knees are at a right angle.

As you slide down, lift your arms in front of you until they are parallel to your shoulders. Keep your back against the wall and hold the position for five counts. Slide back up the wall and lower your arms. Repeat three times.

Variation:

You may use two- or three-pound weights with this exercise. Add small circles with your arms in front of you at shoulder height while in the squat position, with or without weights.

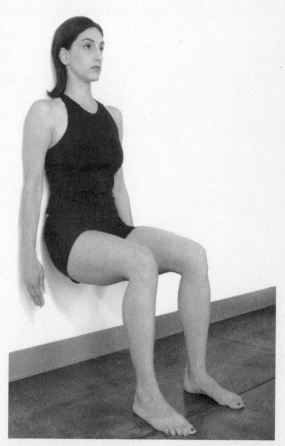

Wall: Squat

Legs

Your legs may already be strong from carrying the extra weight during pregnancy, but now we want to work on lengthening the muscles, making them long, lean, and lovely.

Single Straight Leg

PURPOSE: **Stretch the legs while strengthening the abs.**

Lying on your back, bring your head up and chin to chest. Keeping your right leg straight, raise it toward your body and reach for your right calf with both hands. Keep your shoulders pressed down to the mat. Raise your left leg off the mat a few inches as you gently pull your right leg into your body, feeling the stretch in your hamstring. Alternate legs by scissoring them through the air and pull your left leg into your body. Repeat ten times and do five sets.

Modification:

If you have lower back pain, keep your extended leg higher off the mat.

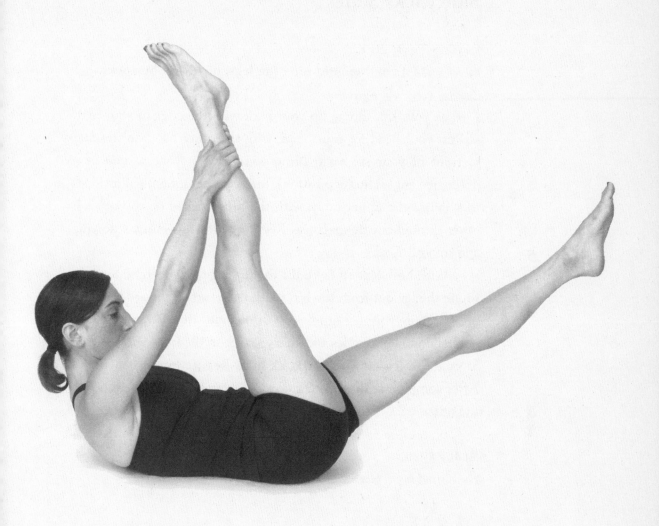

Single Straight Leg

Side Kicks Series

FRONT/BACK

PURPOSE: Lengthen and tone the legs, hips, and buttocks.

Lie on your side, lining up your back with the edge of your mat. Rest your head on your hand, with the other hand on the mat in front of your stomach. Bring your legs in front of you at a 45-degree angle (home position). Engage your abdominal muscles to stabilize the upper body, with the hips stacked on top of each other throughout the exercise. Keep your leg movements flowing and smooth.

With both legs straight, lift the top leg to hip height. Slightly rotate the leg out from the hip (with knee turned toward the ceiling), keeping your leg hip height throughout the exercise. Engage your abdominal muscles and kick your leg to the front with energy. Stretch the leg long on the back kick. Repeat five to ten times. After completing these four side kicks exercises, turn over and do the other leg.

Modification:

For a tired neck, place your head on an outstretched arm.

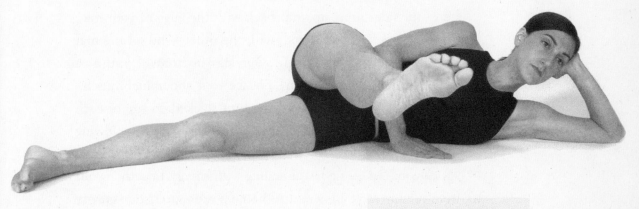

Side Kicks: Front/Back 1

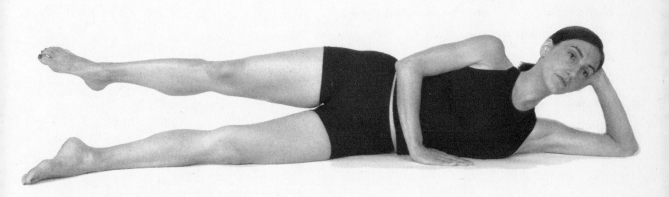

Side Kicks: Front/Back 2

UP/DOWN

PURPOSE: **Lengthen the legs and slim the hips, buttocks, and thighs.**

Lie on your side, lining up your back with the edge of your mat. Rest your head on your hand, with the other hand on the mat in front of your stomach. Bring your legs in front of you at a 45-degree angle (home position). Engage your abdominal muscles to stabilize the upper body, with the hips stacked on top of each other throughout the exercise. Keep your leg movements flowing and smooth.

Kick your top leg up to the ceiling with energy. Lengthen your leg from the hip as you lower it to home position, resisting gravity with your inner thigh. Repeat five times.

C-Section Modification:

Keep your leg movements small and controlled until you are completely pain-free around your stitches.

Modification:

For a tired neck, place your head on an outstretched arm.

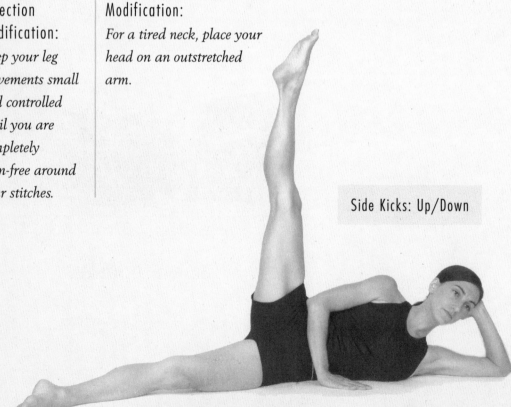

Side Kicks: Up/Down

SMALL CIRCLES

PURPOSE: **Work the hips and outer thighs.**

Lie on your side, lining up your back with the edge of your mat. Rest your head on your hand, with the other hand on the mat in front of your stomach. Bring your legs in front of you at a 45-degree angle (home position). Engage your abdominal muscles to stabilize the upper body, with the hips stacked on top of each other throughout the exercise. Keep your leg movements flowing and smooth.

Starting with your top leg at hip height and slightly turned out, make small circles with your whole leg, not just the foot. Lengthen the leg out of the hip. Repeat five times, then reverse the circles.

Modification:

For a tired neck, place your head on an outstretched arm.

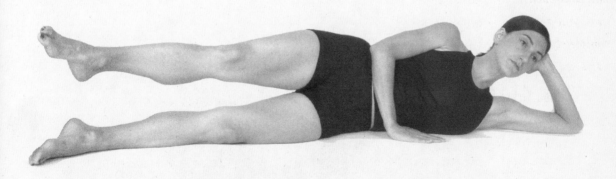

Side Kicks: Small Circles

BICYCLE

PURPOSE: Strengthen and stretch the hips, buttocks, and legs.

Lie on your side, lining up your back with the edge of your mat. Rest your head on your hand, with the other hand on the mat in front of your stomach. Bring your legs in front of you at a 45-degree angle (home position). Engage your abdominal muscles to stabilize the upper body, with the hips stacked on top of each other throughout the exercise. Keep your leg movements flowing and smooth.

Lift your top leg up to hip height. Kick your leg forward, bend your knee, take your bent leg back, then extend it long to home position. Extend your leg long in back and feel a good stretch. Repeat three times, then reverse the movement and bicycle backward.

Modification:

For a tired neck, place your head on an outstretched arm.

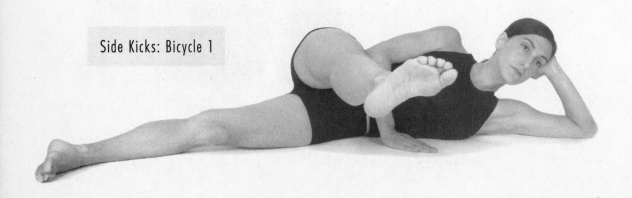

Side Kicks: Bicycle 1

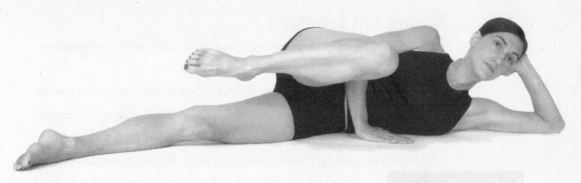

Side Kicks: Bicycle 1

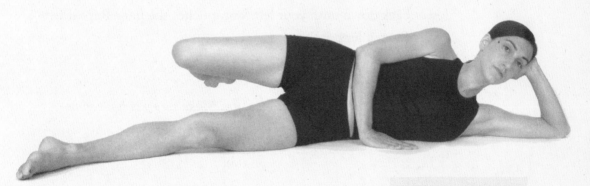

Side Kicks: Bicycle 3

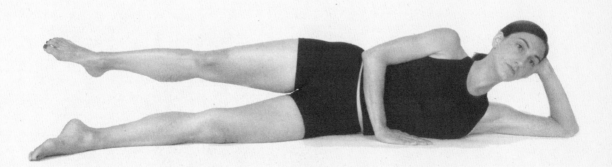

Side Kicks: Bicycle 4

Going Up Front

PURPOSE: Strengthen the legs and butt and improve balance.

Stand in front of a footstool or low and stable chair. Raise your right leg and place your foot flat on the stool. Your knee should be bent at a right angle, with your thigh parallel to the floor. Your right knee should not bend over your toes. Raise your arms out to your sides and slightly round your elbows, keeping them soft. Engage your abdominal muscles to help keep your balance. Stand up on your right leg, lengthening your left leg behind you. Gently lower back down until your left foot touches the floor. Repeat five times. Switch legs.

Modification:

This exercise can also be done on stairs. Make sure you have something to hold on to in case you lose your balance.

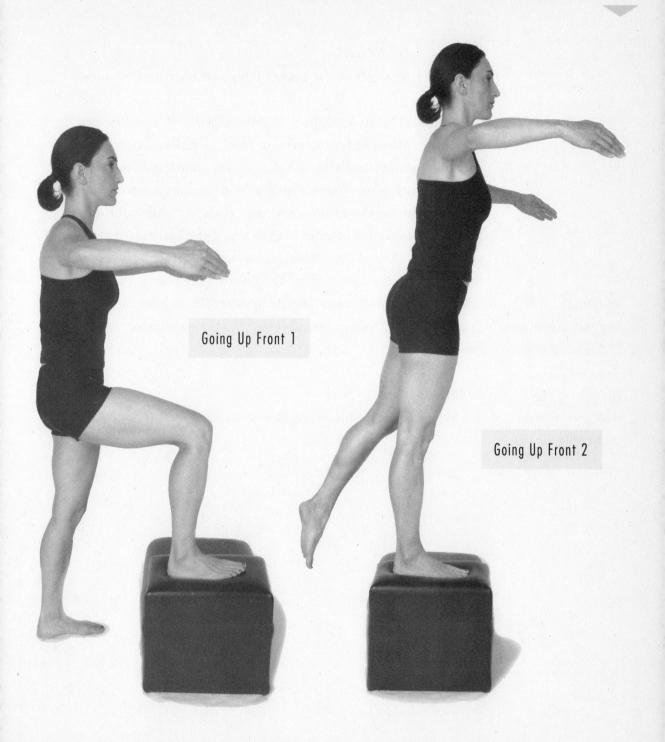

Going Up Front 1

Going Up Front 2

Pliés

PURPOSE: **Strengthen the inner thighs and butt.**

Stand with your legs apart, slightly wider than shoulder distance, with your feet turned out from your hips. Extend your arms to the sides with elbows soft, keeping your shoulders down and relaxed. Engage your abdominal muscles and, keeping your torso upright, bend your knees so they point out over your toes. Bend as deeply as is comfortable, feeling a good stretch through your thighs. Do not bend your knees past the point where your thighs are parallel to the floor. Also ensure that your knees don't roll in and that your torso remains upright. Throughout the bend, squeeze your bottom and stand up to the starting position. Repeat ten times.

Modification:

You may hold on to the back of a chair to stabilize yourself.

Variation:

You may add weights to this exercise by doing the Zip Up (page 114) with your arms while performing the Pliés.

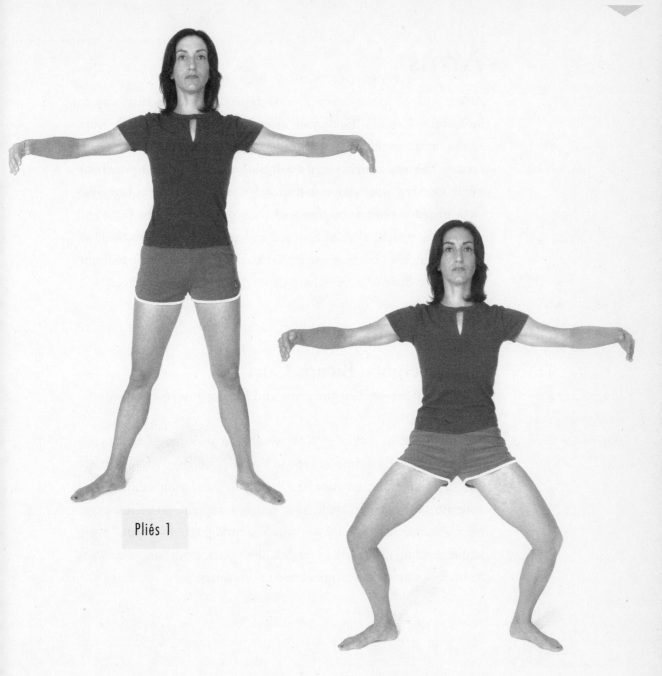

Pliés 1

Pliés 2

Arms

Along with proper posture, having toned arms is an easy way to look better faster. After all, your arms are fairly strong already from all the lifting you do each day, so to tone them, do the following exercises. The arm weights series will tone your arms and upper back while working your abdominal muscles in a standing position. Use two- or three-pound weights and always keep your abs tight and your body weight shifted forward and up with an open chest so you do not lean back or arch your back. Lengthen your tailbone toward the floor while reaching through the top of your head.

Arm Weights: Biceps Curl

PURPOSE: **Strengthen the arms and improve postural strength.**

Stand in Pilates stance. With weights in your hands, bring your arms directly in front of you at shoulder height with palms facing up. Inhale. Engage your biceps as you bend your elbows until your arms form a right angle. Your weights are light so you must create resistance with your own muscles. Straighten your arms again while resisting against the weights like you are pushing your arms through water. Exhale. Repeat five to ten times.

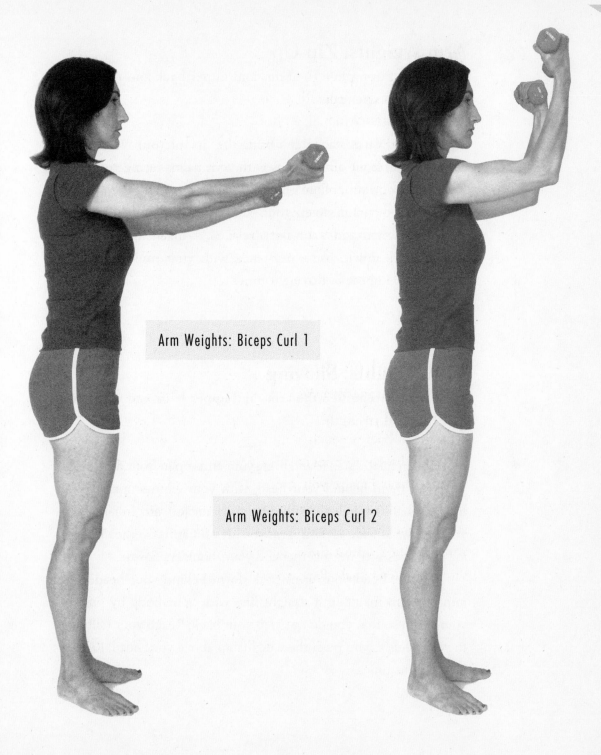

Arm Weights: Biceps Curl 1

Arm Weights: Biceps Curl 2

Arm Weights: Zip Up

PURPOSE: **Strengthen the arms and upper back and improve postural strength.**

Stand in Pilates stance and bring the tips of your weights together in front of your hips with your palms facing your legs. Inhale and bend your elbows out to the sides as you lift the weights up toward your chin. Keep your elbows above your wrists, your shoulders down, and your neck relaxed. Exhale and push the weights back down, using resistance with your muscles against the weights. Repeat five to eight times.

Arm Weights: Shaving

PURPOSE: **Strengthen the arms and upper back and improve postural strength.**

Stand in Pilates stance and bring your arms up in front of you and bend them behind your head, with your elbows open to the sides and hands/weights together, palms facing forward. Inhale. Keep your elbows as wide as possible as you lift your arms overhead, keeping the hands/weights together and your shoulders down.

Exhale. Bend your arms back down behind your head. It is important to maintain a straight line with your body by pulling your abs in so that you do not arch your back. Reach your tailbone to your heels as you push the weights up above your head. Repeat five to eight times.

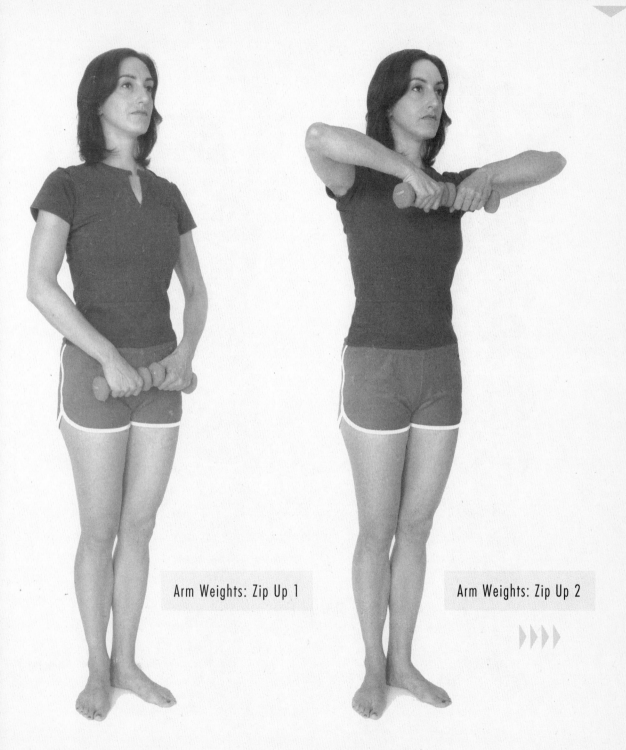

Arm Weights: Zip Up 1

Arm Weights: Zip Up 2

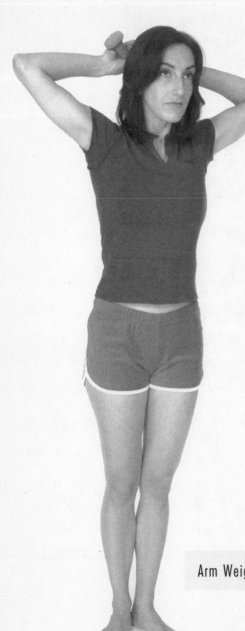

Arm Weights: Shaving 1

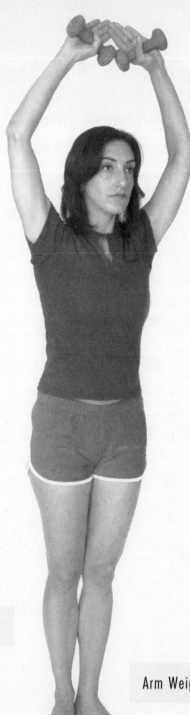

Arm Weights: Shaving 2

Arm Weights: Reverse Curl

PURPOSE: **Strengthen the triceps and improve postural strength.**

Stand in Pilates stance. Holding a weight in each hand, place your hands next to your ribs with your palms facing in and your elbows pointing behind you. Engage your abdominal muscles and maintain a long neck and spine. Squeeze your triceps as you straighten your arms out behind you, moving your forearms from the elbows and keeping your upper arm stable. Repeat five to eight times.

Arm Weights: Reverse Curl 1

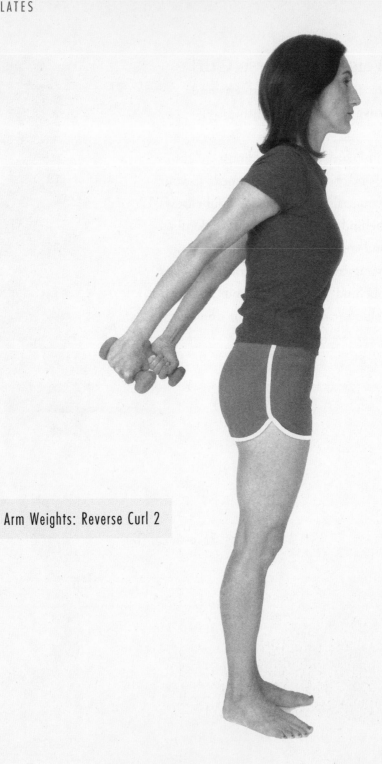

Arm Weights: Reverse Curl 2

Backward Arms

PURPOSE: **Strengthen upper back, arms, and abs.**

Sitting on the front edge of a stable chair, place your arms at your sides with the heel of your hands on the front edge of the chair. Keep your feet hip-distance apart and your wrists aligned with your shoulders. Your fingers should be pointing forward.

Use your arms to lift your butt slightly off the chair as you engage your abdominal muscles. Move your body forward slightly and bend your elbows back to lower your body toward the floor until your elbows make a right angle. Pull your shoulder blades down and together and keep your chest open. Press your body back up to starting position, and be careful not to lock your elbows. Repeat five times without sitting down. When you become stronger, work up to ten repetitions, doing three sets.

Modification:

This exercise can also be done on a footstool, or on stairs. If you have any shoulder pain, leave this exercise out until you become stronger.

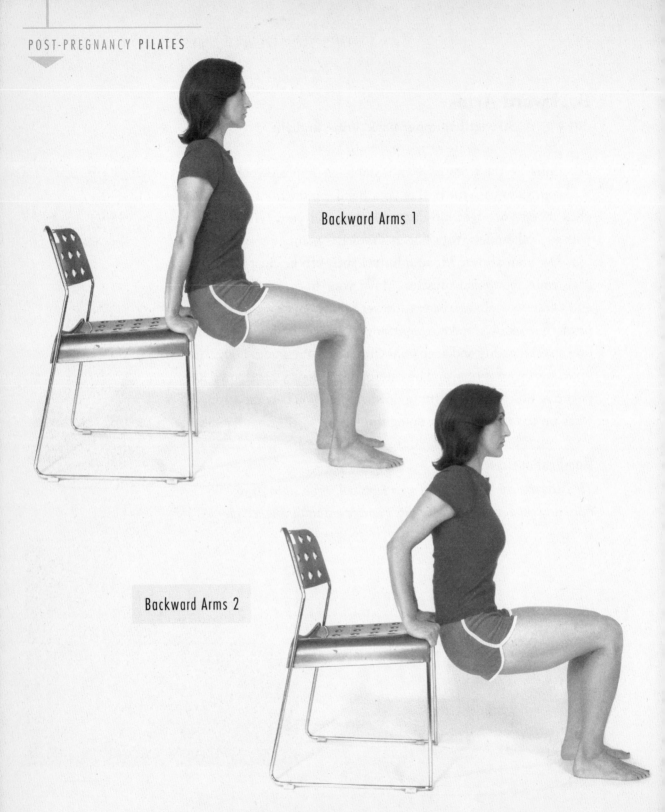

Backward Arms 1

Backward Arms 2

Wall: Push-ups

PURPOSE: Strengthen the upper body and
    abs; can be done as an alternative to
    regular Push-ups (page 200).

Stand an arm's distance away from a wall
and place your hands at shoulder height
against the wall. Inhale. Engage your abdominal muscles and lean into the wall, bending
your elbows toward the floor, then exhale and
gently push yourself away. Remember to keep
your body in a straight line and focus on your
core in addition to your arms. Look straight in
front of you to keep your neck in line. Repeat
ten times with control. Work up to three sets,
and when you are strong enough, do Pilates
push-ups on the mat.

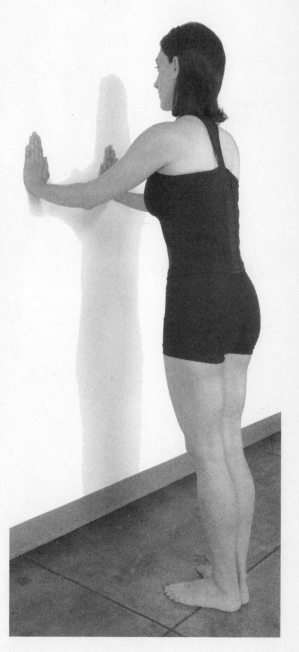

Wall: Push-ups 1

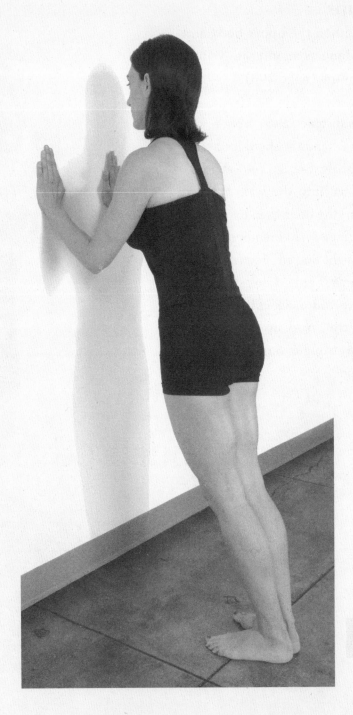

Wall: Push-ups 2

6

Mommy Aches and Pains:

Pilates Solutions to Healing Your Body

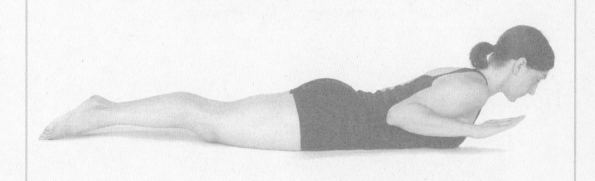

Even if you had an easy pregnancy, a quick and pain-free labor and delivery, and have tons of helpers at your disposal (yeah, like you are living in the movies), you are still going to be exhausted after giving birth. And this exhaustion can cause you to develop bad postural habits, leading to lower back pain and neck tension, which gets in the way of enjoying your baby and getting your life back.

Proper breathing techniques are very important during exercise and also in your daily activities. Focused breathing can release tension in your body, help relieve headaches, and increase endurance. Think about times when you became angry but stopped to take a breath to avoid blowing up. Or when you had a massage and the therapist told you to breathe through a particularly painful spot. Or when you gave birth—your breath helped you manage the pain and deliver your baby!

This chapter includes exercises that target specific complaints that new moms have. Most of these exercises are included in the three recovery workouts and the Mommy Maintenance Workout, so you will experience their pain-relieving benefits no matter which workout you do. But when you wake up one day with nagging neck pain or persistent back pain, you may want to take some time to work it out through these individual programs.

Tip: Time for yourself is essential—not self-indulgent.

Neck Pain

Neck pain can develop as a result of many of your new-mom movements—hunching over your baby while feeding him, carrying a heavy diaper bag, toting the baby in a front carrier, or even looking down and gazing lovingly into the eyes of your little one. I came to this unfortunate realization when I found that, after being home with my son most of the time, I was always looking down in order to talk to him, since he was the shortest—and only—guy around. I had to adjust our conversation positions to save my neck and shoulders.

Because one of the biggest contributors to neck pain is your posture while feeding your baby, make sure to find a good feeding position, with your feet supported. Keep your head and neck aligned on top of your shoulders. Relax your body, keeping your shoulders free of tension; place a cushion behind your back and don't lean forward.

To treat back and shoulder pain that develops despite your perfect feeding posture, I of course recommend having your partner give you massages on demand and treating yourself to a professional massage occasionally. But for long-term relief, you need to strengthen your neck and learn ways to prevent future problems.

Neck Turns

PURPOSE: Stretch the neck muscles, promote flexibility of the upper spine, and release neck and upper back tension.

Standing or sitting in an upright position, turn your head and look to one side and hold for five counts. Make sure your shoulders stay down and relaxed. Turn your head back to center, then look to the other side, holding for five counts. Repeat three times each side, alternating sides.

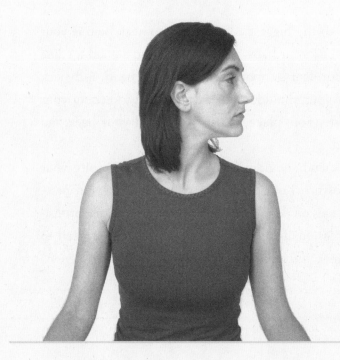

Neck Turns

Neck Circles

PURPOSE: Stretch the neck muscles, promote flexibility of the upper spine, and release neck and upper back tension.

Standing or sitting in an upright position, roll your head by inclining your ear toward your shoulder, then rolling your chin toward your chest, to the other ear, and up. Do not allow your head to rotate to the back, but instead pass through center with your head erect. Always keep your shoulders down. Repeat two times in each direction.

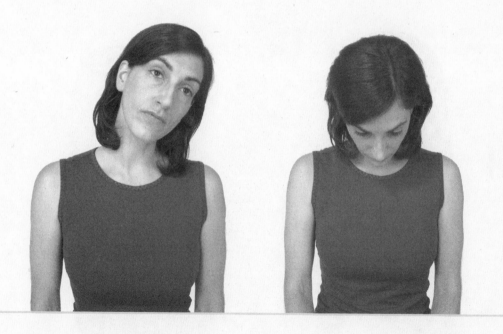

Neck Circles 1 and 2

Shoulder Rolls

PURPOSE: Promote relaxation, increase flexibility in the shoulders, and improve circulation.

Begin by standing or sitting in an upright position. Engage your abs while keeping the rest of your body relaxed. Roll your shoulders up, then forward and downward, making big circles. Be sure to end each movement with your shoulders back and your chest open. Repeat five times. Reverse the direction by rolling your shoulders backward, again ending with your chest open and your shoulders back.

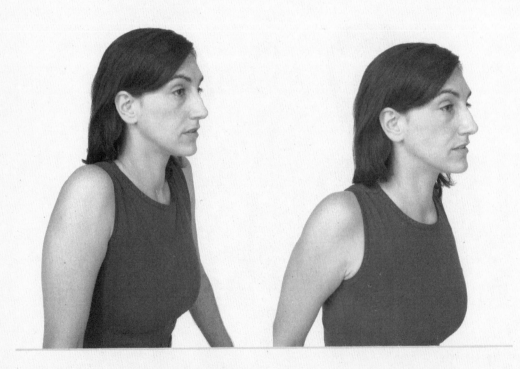

Shoulder Rolls 1 and 2

Neck Exercise

PURPOSE: Strengthen the neck.

Begin in either a standing or a seated position. Keep your neck long, shoulders relaxed, and body upright. Overlap your hands at the back of your neck, right at the base of your head. With your elbows pointing out to the sides, gently press your head into your hands. Hold for ten counts. Repeat three times. Over time, gradually increase the duration of the hold to twenty, and then thirty counts.

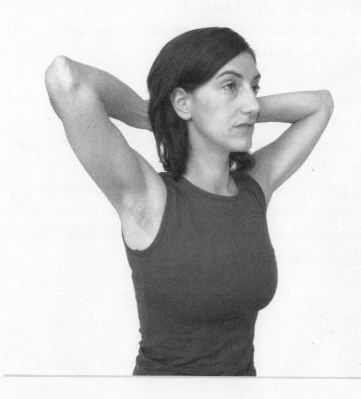

Neck Exercise

Upper Back Pain

Upper back pain can come from hunching forward due to "pregnant posture," which is standing with your shoulders pulled forward in response to the excess weight being carried on the front of your body. This can weaken your upper back, strain your shoulders, and cause tension in the neck.

Arm Weights: The Hug

PURPOSE: Strengthen the arms, chest, and upper back, and improve postural strength.

With a weight in each hand, stand in Pilates stance. Raise your arms to the sides at shoulder height. Slightly round your elbows, keeping them soft, so that your arms curl in like you are hugging a large ball. Hold the weights almost perpendicular to the floor, tilted slightly inward. Inhale and bring your arms together, engaging your chest muscles while keeping your abs in. Exhale as you open your arms, pulling your shoulder blades together. Repeat five to eight times.

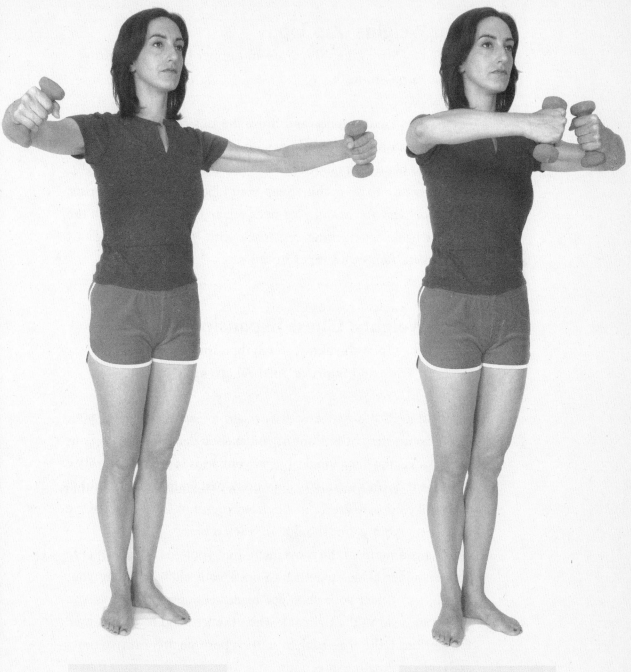

Arm Weights: The Hug 1

Arm Weights: The Hug 2

Arm Weights: Zip Up

PURPOSE: Strengthen the arms and upper back and improve postural strength.

Stand in Pilates stance and bring the tips of your weights together in front of your hips with your palms facing your legs. Inhale and bend your elbows out to the sides as you lift the weights all the way up to your chin. Keep your elbows above your wrists, your shoulders down, and your neck relaxed. Exhale and push the weights back down, using resistance with your muscles against the weights. Repeat five to eight times.

Arm Weights: Chest Expansion

PURPOSE: Open the chest, strengthen the upper back and arms, and improve postural strength.

Stand in Pilates stance with a weight in each hand. Bring your arms up straight in front of you at shoulder height, with your palms facing the floor. Inhale. Lower your arms in a slow, controlled movement down the front of your body, past your hips, and behind you until your arms are 12 inches from your butt. At the end of the movement, your palms should face each other.

As you perform the movement, pull your abs in and squeeze your shoulder blades together to open your chest. Holding your breath, try to feel your shoulder blades coming together as you turn your head to the right side, then the left, and back to center. Exhale. Reach the arms back to starting position. Repeat two times each side, alternating directions.

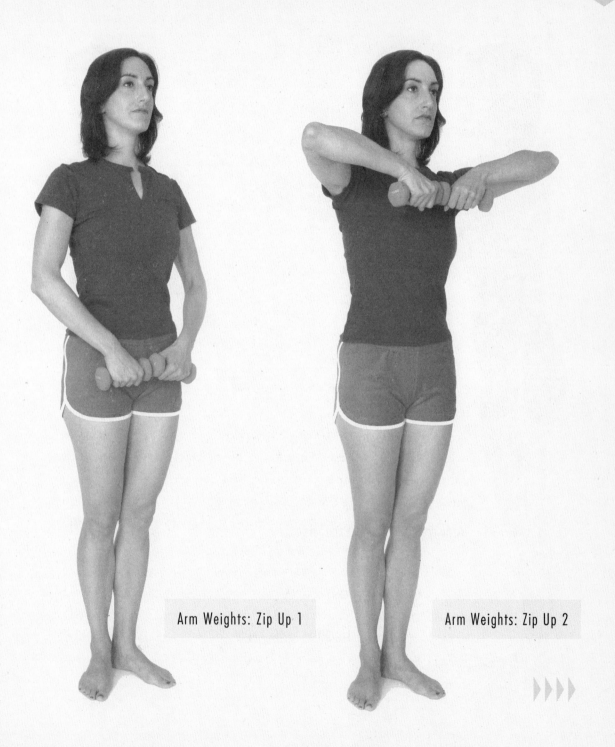

Arm Weights: Zip Up 1

Arm Weights: Zip Up 2

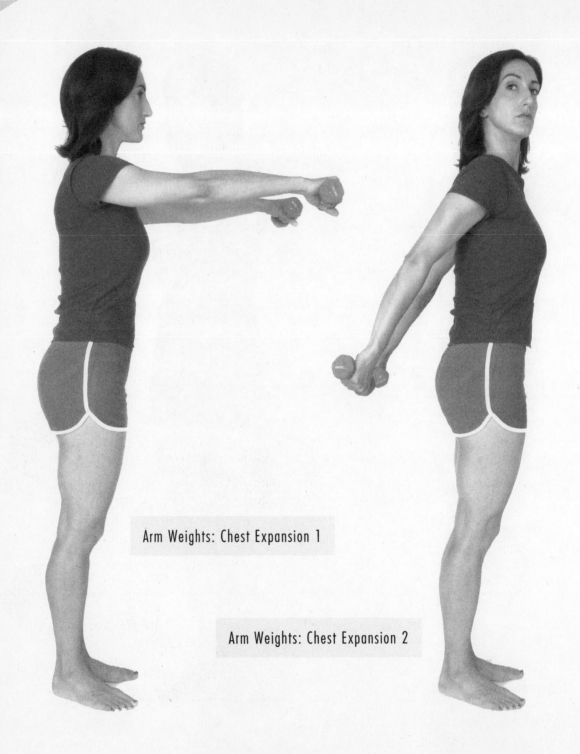

Arm Weights: Chest Expansion 1

Arm Weights: Chest Expansion 2

Upper Body Lift

PURPOSE: Strengthen the upper back.

Lie on your stomach with legs together and your face down on the mat. Place your palms down next to your shoulders and bend your elbows so that your arms rest alongside your body. Keeping your shoulder blades reaching down your back and abdominal muscles lifted, gently raise your upper body and hands off the mat a few inches and hold for five counts. Do not use your hands to press yourself off the mat. Slowly release. Remember to reach through the top of your head, lengthening your body as opposed to lifting your head up.

Modification:

This exercise may be uncomfortable at first if your breasts are sore or engorged or if you have lower back pain. If that is the case, skip it for now.

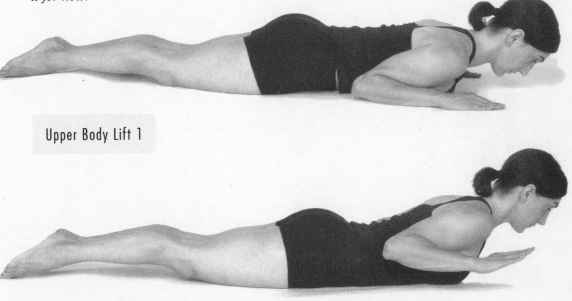

Upper Body Lift 1

Upper Body Lift 2

135

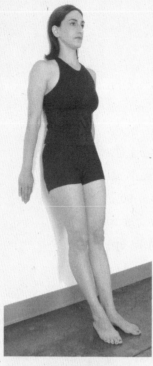

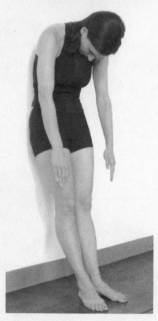

Wall: Rolling Down

PURPOSE: **Strengthen the abs, stretch the back, and promote relaxation.**

Standing with your back against a wall, bring your chin to your chest. Relax your shoulders and place your arms at your sides. Keeping your stomach lifted and pressed into your spine, start to peel your back off the wall beginning with the shoulders, removing one vertebra at a time. Roll down to your waist while pressing your lower back against the wall by keeping your abs pulled in tight. Your fingers will likely be at knee level.

Maintain stillness in your body, feeling gravity pull you down. Let your arms hang heavy and make a few tiny, loose, effortless circles in one direction. Then reverse the direction of the circles. Try to let your arms stop moving on their own.

Pull your abs in and up, slowly rolling back up the wall, pressing each vertebra into the wall until you are standing erect.

Wall: Rolling Down 1 and 2

Lower Back Pain

Lower back pain is often caused by tight hip flexors that result from sitting for long periods of time. It can also be caused by the excess weight you carried in front throughout pregnancy, and from bending over to pick things up. Pregnancy hormones soften muscle tissue so your joints are not well supported. It is therefore important to build abdominal strength to support your lower back, as well as relieve tension in this area.

Tummy Tightener

PURPOSE: **Wake up and strengthen the abdominal muscles and the back.**

Lie on your back with knees bent and feet flat on the floor hip-distance apart. Relax your chest and ribs. Inhale. Pull your abdominal muscles in by imagining you are trying to reach your belly button to your spine, and feel your abs tighten. Hold for five counts. Exhale. Repeat five times.

Do not tense your upper back or push with your feet. Once you have the hang of this, you can do it sitting or standing anywhere you please. Work your way up to holding the movement for ten counts.

Pelvic Curl

PURPOSE: Release tension in the lower back by lengthening the spine; strengthen the abdominal muscles and pelvic floor.

Lying flat on your back, bend your knees and keep your feet on the ground, hip-distance apart. Completely relax your upper body, reaching your shoulder blades down your back. Engage (or imagine engaging) your lower abdominal muscles by pulling them in. This subtle movement will result in your tailbone reaching away from your body and your spine lengthening.

Hold for ten counts. Release slowly without creating tension in your upper back. Repeat three times in the beginning, working your way up to five, and later ten. Be sure to breathe normally. When you have mastered the Pelvic Curl, add a Kegel (page 18) while you hold the curl. Release the Kegel hold as you release the curl position.

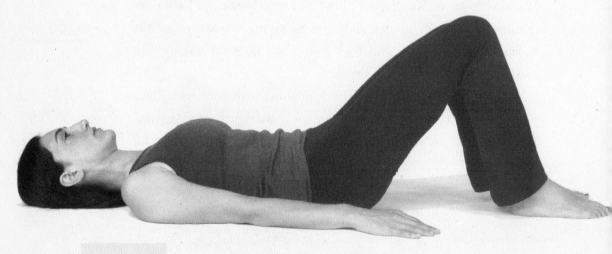

Pelvic Curl

138

Hundred *(modified)*

PURPOSE: **Strengthen the abdominal muscles and increase endurance by focusing on breathing; a warm-up for the exercises that follow.**

Begin by lying on your back. Raise your legs straight up toward the ceiling, then bend your knees at a right angle so that your calves are parallel to the floor. Keep your arms down by your sides. Take one deep inhalation through the nose for five counts, then one full exhalation through the mouth for five counts. This is one set. Begin pumping your straight arms up and down, about 4–6 inches off the floor.

Once you have mastered the breathing, lift your head, and bring your chin toward your chest. As you become stronger, extend your legs straight up toward the ceiling. Do ten sets.

Hundred

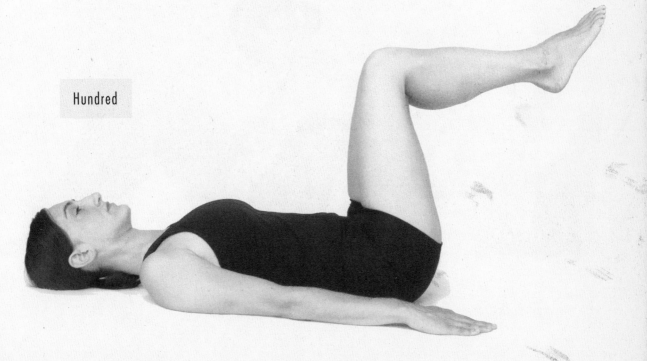

Roll Back

PURPOSE: **Strengthen the abs and stretch and open the lower back.**

Sit upright with your knees bent and your feet on the floor hip-distance apart. Lightly hold on to the back of your thighs with your hands. Pull your abdominal muscles in and let your shoulders relax forward. Roll backward by pulling your stomach in so that your tailbone tucks under and tilts forward. Roll down until your waistband touches the mat and hold for five counts. Come back up to a sitting position using only your abdominal muscles, not your arms. As you get stronger, you may roll back even farther. Repeat five times.

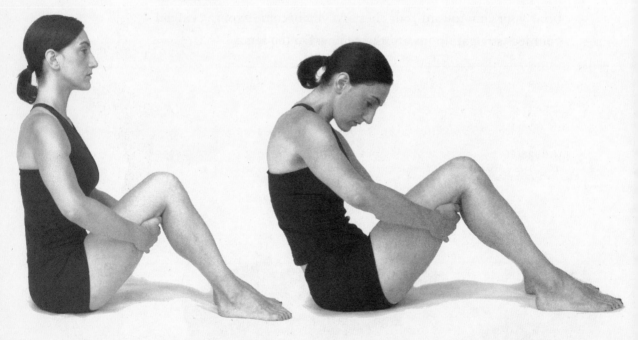

Roll Back 1   Roll Back 2

Wall: Rolling Down

PURPOSE: Strengthen the abs, stretch the back,
and promote relaxation.

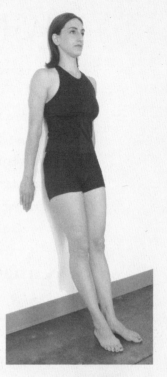

Standing with your back against a wall, bring your
chin to your chest. Relax your shoulders and
place your arms at your sides. Keeping your stomach
lifted and pressed into your spine, start to peel your
back off the wall beginning with the shoulders, removing one vertebra at a time. Roll down to your
waist while pressing your lower back against the wall
by keeping your abs pulled in tight. Your fingers will
likely be at knee level.

Maintain stillness in your body, feeling gravity
pull you down. Let your arms hang heavy and make a
few tiny, loose, effortless circles in one direction. Then
reverse the direction of the circles. Try to let your
arms stop moving on their own.

Pull your abs in and up, slowly rolling back up
the wall, pressing each vertebra into the wall until
you are standing erect.

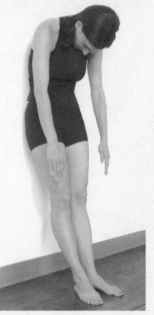

Wall: Rolling Down 1 and 2

141

Wrist Pain

Some women develop carpal tunnel syndrome during pregnancy from fluid retention and swelling, which affects blood flow due to compression of the median nerve of the wrist. This may sound strange, but some moms experience this problem from their baby's butt resting on their forearm for long periods of time. No kidding. I had a girlfriend who had to get physical therapy for this. So move your baby around!

Castanets

PURPOSE: **Strengthen and stretch the hands and fingers; prevent/help to rehabilitate carpal tunnel syndrome.**

Standing in Pilates stance, raise your arms in front of you to shoulder height, palms facing each other. Slightly bend your elbows to the sides. Tap each finger to the thumb on the same hand ten times. (Thumb to pointer 1–2–3–4–5 . . . , thumb to middle 1–2–3–4–5 . . . , etc.) Then reverse, starting with thumb to pinkie. Repeat two times in each direction.

Wrist Stretches

PURPOSE: **Stretch the wrist.**

In a standing or seated position, extend your right arm in front of you at shoulder height. Point your fingers down and your palm away from your body. Grasp your right fingers with your left hand and gently pull the fingers toward you. Keep your palm firm and straight. Hold for ten counts. Do the same on the left hand. Repeat two times. You can also do this exercise with fingers pointing up to the ceiling.

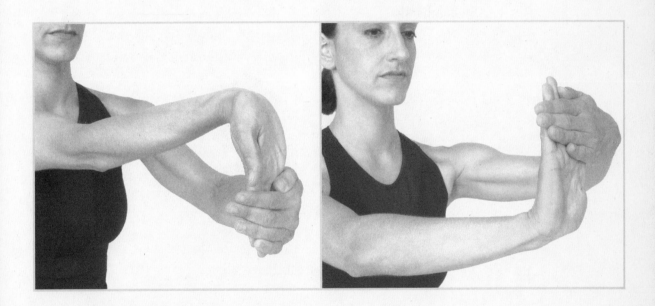

Wrist Stretches 1 and 2

143

Arm Weights: Wrist Raises

PURPOSE: Strengthen the wrists and prevent/help
to rehabilitate carpal tunnel syndrome.

Holding a 2-pound weight, stand with feet in Pilates stance and bend your arm at a right angle at your side, keeping your elbow pointing back close to your ribs and your palm facing up. Bend your wrist up, bringing your weight toward you, without moving your arm. Then release it back to starting position. This is a wrist-strengthening exercise so focus only on the movement of your wrist by stabilizing your arm against your body. Repeat five times. Switch hands.

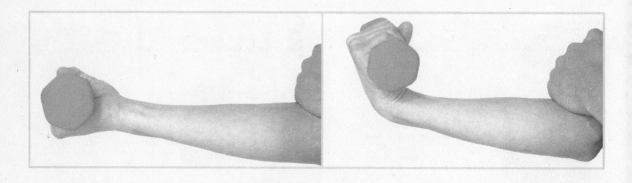

Arm Weights: Wrist Raises 1 and 2

7

Mommy Maintenance:
Developing the Body You Deserve

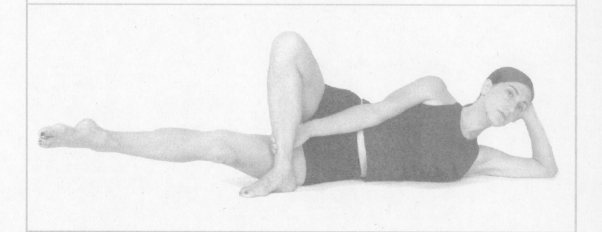

By the time Ches was a few months old, I was completely addicted to my Pilates classes and loved the energy they gave me, not to mention my body, which was, I must say, lean and mean. As soon as my husband came home from work in the evening, I dashed out to get to class on time. This was my twice-a-week program, supplemented by whatever I could do at home, which, honestly, was difficult because I didn't have a book to help me learn the exercises. This book is intended to make it easier for you to stay focused and on track at home.

So here it is—everything you need to get a complete workout at home. Following this program will firm you up, slim you down, and energize you for the most important job you face: being a mom.

Many of the floor exercises are performed with your head up and chin toward your chest so that you are looking at your belly. If you have any neck discomfort or tension, you may keep your head down during the exercises. The "variation" suggestion assumes you have enough strength to take the exercise to the next level.

Tummy Tightener *(Beginner)*

PURPOSE: **Wake up and strengthen the abdominal muscles and the back.**

Lie on your back with knees bent and feet flat on the floor hip-distance apart. Relax your chest and ribs. Inhale. Pull your abdominal muscles in by imagining you are trying to reach your belly button to your spine, and feel your abs tighten. Hold for five counts. Exhale. Repeat five times.

Do not tense your upper back or push with your feet. Once you have the hang of this, you can do it sitting or standing anywhere you please. Work your way up to holding the movement for ten counts.

Hundred *(Beginner)*

PURPOSE: Strengthen the abdominal muscles and increase endurance by focusing on breathing; a warm-up for the exercises that follow.

Begin by lying on your back. Raise your legs straight up toward the ceiling so that your body and legs form a 90-degree angle. Keep your arms down by your sides. Take one deep inhalation through the nose for five counts, then one full exhalation through the mouth for five counts. This is one set. Begin pumping your straight arms up and down, about 4–6 inches off the floor. Once you have mastered the breathing, lift your head and bring your chin toward your chest. Do ten sets.

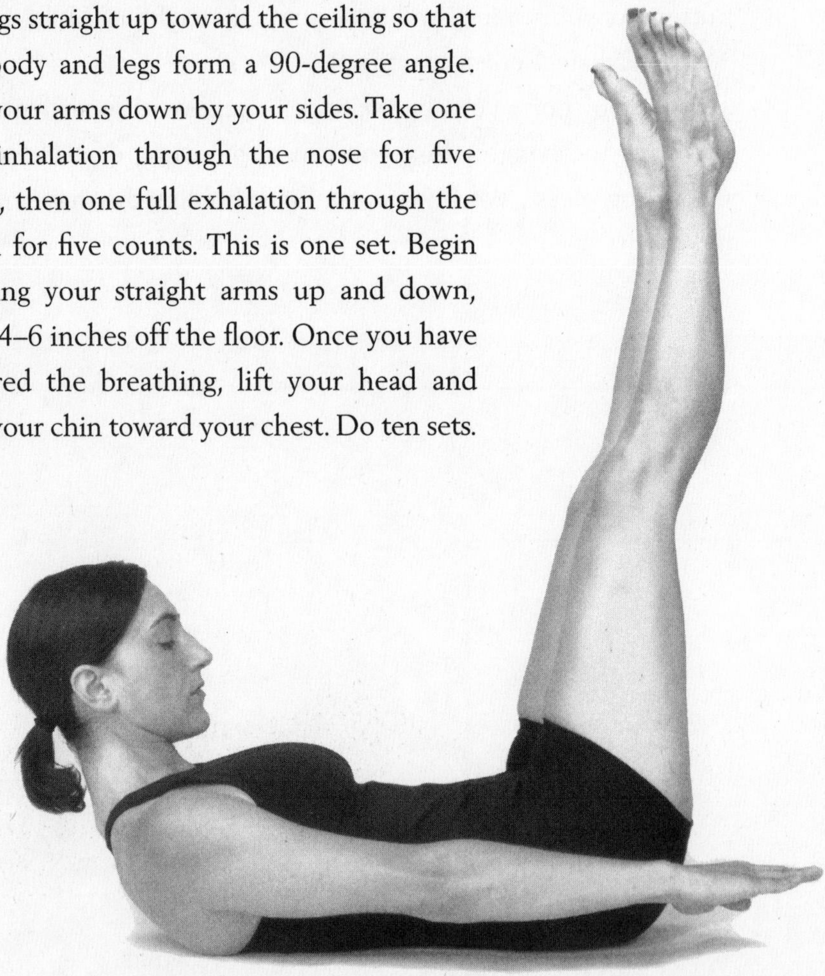

Hundred

148

Baby Steps/C-Section Modification:

Place your feet on the floor with knees bent, bring your head up, and pump your arms while breathing as stated above. Alternatively, you may keep your knees bent at a right angle with head down (for a tired or tense neck) or up.

Variation:

As your abdominal muscles get even stronger, try lowering your legs toward the floor, but make sure to maintain your lower back on the floor.

Hundred (Modified)

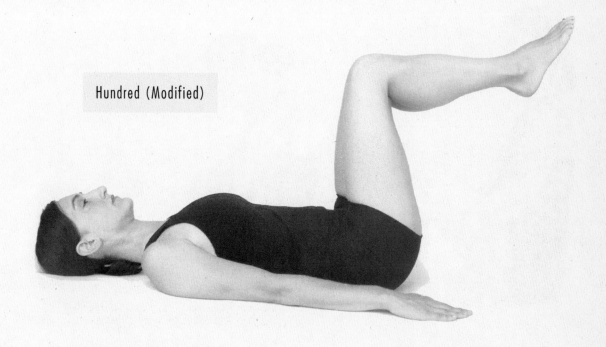

Roll Back *(Beginner)*

PURPOSE: Strengthen the abs and stretch and open the lower back; can be used as a preparation for the Roll Up (opposite).

Sit upright with your knees bent and your feet on the floor hip-distance apart. Lightly hold on to the back of your thighs with your hands. Pull your abdominal muscles in and let your shoulders relax forward. Roll backward by pulling your stomach in so that your tailbone tucks under and tilts forward. Roll down until your waistband touches the mat and hold for five counts. Come back up to a sitting position using only your abdominal muscles, not your arms. As you get stronger, you may roll back even farther. Repeat five times.

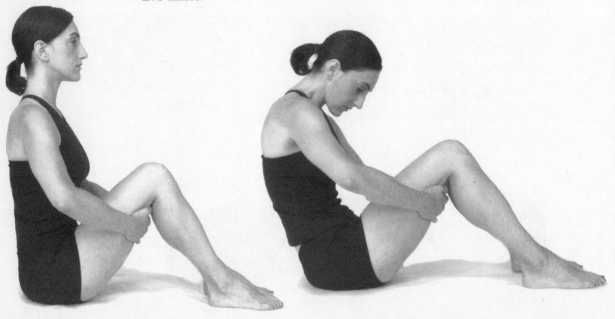

Roll Back (Beginner) 1   Roll Back (Beginner) 2

Roll Up *(Beginner)*

PURPOSE: **Strengthen the abs and stretch the spine
and back of the legs.**

Lie on your back with straight legs and feet in Pilates stance. Extend your arms straight overhead so that they are parallel to your ears, shoulder-width apart. Raise your head and inhale, then lift your arms toward the ceiling and begin rolling up, pulling your abdominal muscles in while reaching arms forward. Exhale as you reach beyond your toes.

Inhale, pull your abs in, and begin to roll back down, trying to touch each vertebra consecutively on the mat until you are lying flat again with arms up by your ears. Exhale as you return to the starting position. Repeat three to five times.

Modification:

Bend your knees slightly and keep your arms by your sides if you cannot roll up smoothly.

C-Section Modification:

Refer to the Roll Back (previous page) until you are well on your way to being healed.

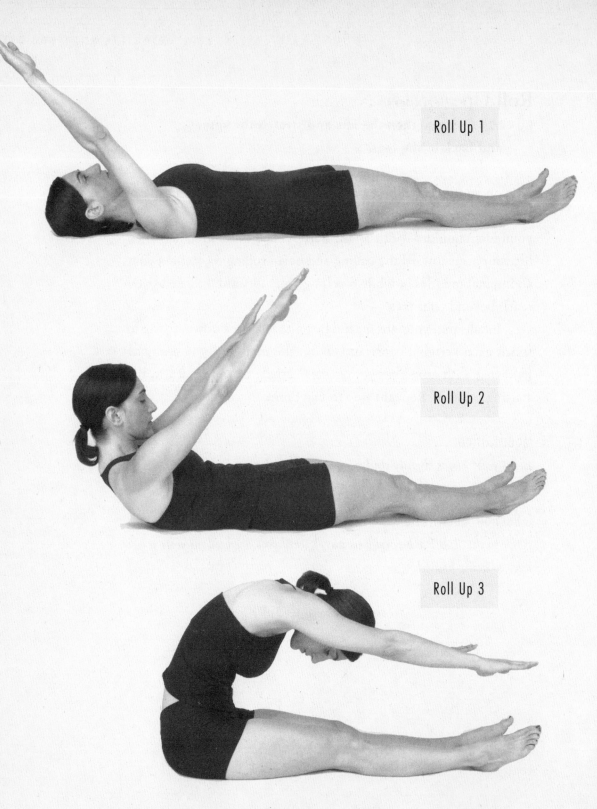

Roll Up 1

Roll Up 2

Roll Up 3

152

Roll Over *(Advanced)*

**PURPOSE: Strengthen the abs and stretch the legs
and lower back.**

Lie on your back with your arms at your sides. Extend your legs straight up to the ceiling, feet in Pilates stance with your toes pointed. Inhale and lift your buttocks up and off the mat by using your abdominal muscles. Lift your legs so that your feet point over your head and behind you until your legs are parallel to the floor, with your toes almost touching the floor above your head.

Exhale. Open your legs shoulder distance apart, flex your feet, and start to slowly roll down your spine, keeping your legs close to your chest. When your tailbone reaches the mat and your legs are at a 90-degree angle, close your legs in Pilates stance and point your toes. Begin and end with your legs straight at a 90-degree angle. Repeat the exercise two more times.

Next, perform the exercise with the position of your feet reversed. Keep your legs open and toes pointed as you roll over, and keep your legs closed and feet flexed as you roll down. Repeat two times.

Variation:

As you become stronger, lower your legs closer to the floor during the roll over.

Roll Over 1

Roll Over 2

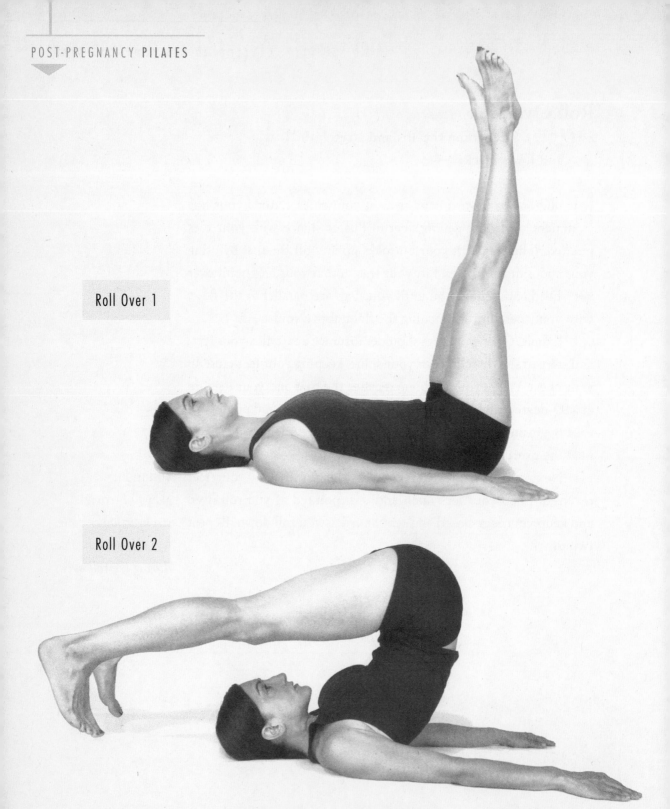

Single Leg Circles *(Beginner)*

PURPOSE: **Strengthen and stabilize the hips and lengthen and trim the legs.**

Lie on your back with arms relaxed at your sides. Keeping your left leg straight, raise your right leg up to the ceiling. Be sure to keep your head down. Slightly rotate your right leg out from the hip, making circles by first crossing over your body with your leg, then down, out to the side, and up. Start and stop the circle with your foot over your nose, the center of your body. Keep your leg loose and your hips anchored to the mat with your abdominal muscles. Repeat five times, then reverse the circles five times.

Modification/
C-Section
Modification:

If you cannot keep your back flat or you feel a strain in your knee, start by doing this exercise with one leg bent, foot on the floor, while making circles with the other leg.

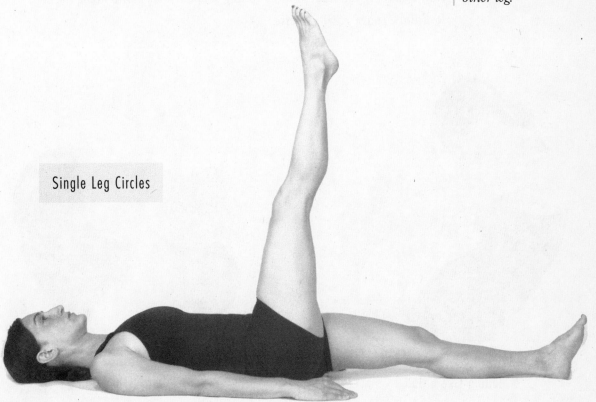

Single Leg Circles

Rolling Like a Ball *(Beginner)*

PURPOSE: **Massage the spine and improve balance.**

In a sitting position, bring your knees close to your chest. Hold on to your ankles and bring your head down to your knees. Lift your feet off the floor. Balance in a tight ball by keeping your feet close to your buttocks and your abs pulled in. Inhale. Roll back onto your shoulder blades and exhale. Roll up to sitting, holding the position by balancing. Avoid rolling on to your neck. Repeat six times.

Modification:

If you have knee pain, hold on to the back of your thighs instead of your ankles. If you have trouble rolling smoothly, keep practicing the Roll Back (page 150) exercise.

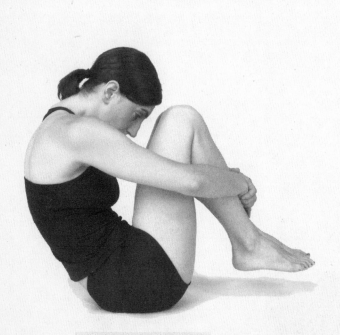

Rolling Like a Ball 1

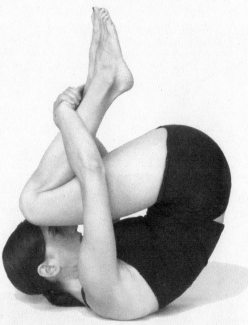

Rolling Like a Ball 2

Single Leg Stretch *(Beginner)*

PURPOSE: **Strengthen the abs and stretch the back of the legs.**

Lying on your back, bend your right knee to your chest. Place your right hand on the right ankle and left hand on right knee. Bring your head up and chin to your chest and lift your left leg at a 45-degree angle to the ground. Remember that this is not just an abdominal exercise but also a stretch for the back of your legs (hamstrings), so be sure to feel the stretch in your right leg.

Switch legs, pulling your left knee into your chest, with your left hand on the left ankle and right hand on left knee. Keep your legs in alignment when bent or straight by directing them down the centerline of your body. Repeat ten times and do five sets.

Modification:

If you have knee pain, place your hands under your knees. If you have lower back pain, keep your legs higher with your heels over your hips.

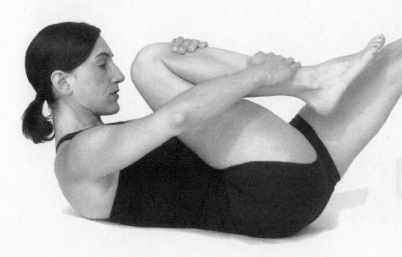

Single Leg Stretch

Double Leg Stretch *(Beginner)*
PURPOSE: Strengthen the abs and stretch the body.

Lying on your back, bring both knees into your chest, holding on to your ankles. Bring your head up and chin toward your chest. Inhale. Raise your arms over your head so they are straight and close to your ears. At the same time, extend your legs straight at a 45-degree angle to the ground.

Circle your arms out to the sides and exhale. Complete the arm circle by reaching for your ankles as you pull your knees back in to your chest. Your legs should stay together throughout the exercise. Repeat five to ten times.

Modification:
If you have knee pain, place your hands under your knees. If you have back pain, raise your legs higher off the mat.

Double Leg Stretch 1

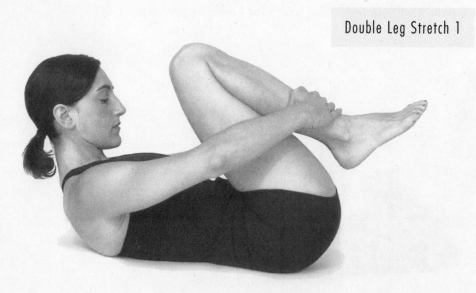

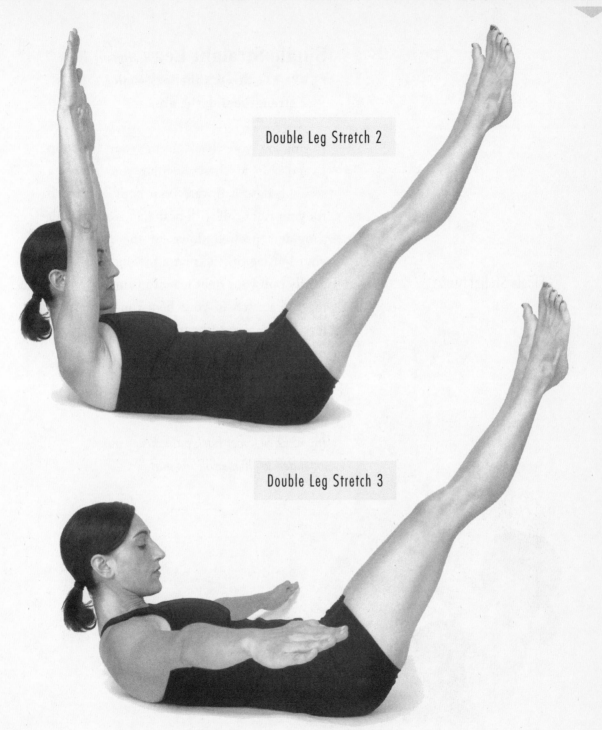

Double Leg Stretch 2

Double Leg Stretch 3

Single Straight Leg *(Intermediate)*

PURPOSE: **Stretch the legs while strengthening the abs.**

Lying on your back, bring your head up and chin to chest. Keeping your right leg straight, raise it toward your body and reach for your right calf with both hands. Keep your shoulders pressed down to the mat. Raise your left leg off the mat a few inches as you gently pull your right leg into your body, feeling the stretch in your hamstring. Alternate legs by scissoring them through the air and pull your left leg into your body. Repeat ten times and do five sets.

Modification:
If you have lower back pain, keep your extended leg higher off the mat.

Single Straight Leg

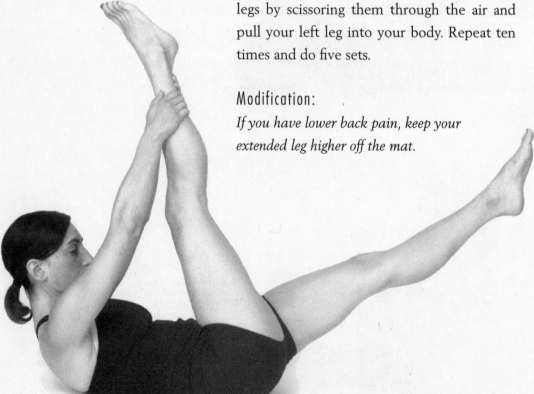

Double Straight Leg *(Intermediate)*
PURPOSE: **Strengthen the lower and upper abs.**

Lying on your back with hands behind your head and elbows pointing out to the sides, bring your head up and chin to chest. Raise your legs straight up until your feet are pointing to the ceiling, keeping them in Pilates stance. Pull your abdominal muscles in, inhale, and lower your legs together. Lower them as close to the mat as you can while keeping your back pressed into the mat. Exhale and bring the legs back up. Repeat five to ten times.

Modification:
If you have lower back pain, keep your legs higher with knees slightly bent and/or place your hands under your buttocks.

C-Section Modification:
Leave this exercise out until you are completely healed.

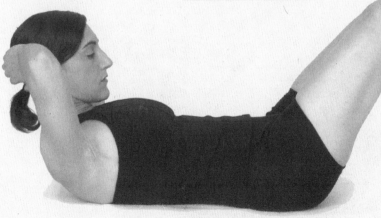

Double Straight Leg

Crisscross (Intermediate)

PURPOSE: Strengthen the oblique muscles and trim the waistline.

Lying on your back with hands behind your head and elbows pointing out to the sides, bring your head up and chin to chest. Slightly lift your upper body by pressing your ribs down and rolling your shoulders off the mat. Inhale. Bend your right knee up to your chest as the left leg extends straight; bring left elbow to right knee and look at your right elbow. Keep both elbows open wide. Stabilize with your abs; only your upper body should twist. Hold for three counts and exhale as you come to center. Inhale again as you switch sides. Do three sets.

Modification/C-Section Modification (see page 73):

Reach your hands in front of you, placing one on top of the other with knees bent and feet flat on the mat hip-distance apart. Using your obliques (side ab muscles), reach up and to the right of your knees. Hold for one count. Then twist and reach to the left of your knees. Try not to rest between sides.

Crisscross

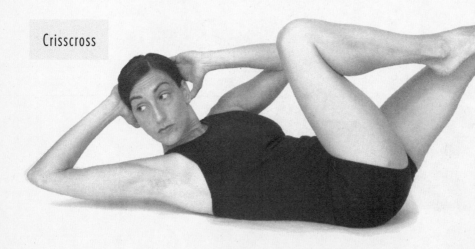

162

Spine Stretch Forward *(Beginner)*

PURPOSE: **Enhance postural strength (abs, back) and stretch the back and the legs.**

Sit up tall with your legs extended to the outer edges of the mat and feet flexed. Reach your arms in front of you, shoulder height and shoulder-width apart. Inhale as you squeeze your buttocks, lift your pelvic floor muscles, and sit up taller. Bring your chin to your chest and reach forward by rolling down your spine. Your stomach should continue lifting, as though you are bending over a big ball. Keep reaching your arms in front of you with relaxed shoulders. Exhale.

Inhale as you start to roll back up, pulling your abs in. Reach your fingers forward as you continue to sit up tall. Keep lifting when you reach the top, then exhale. Repeat three to five times.

Modification:

If you have back or knee pain, bend your knees slightly, or sit on a firm pillow to position your hips slightly higher than your feet.

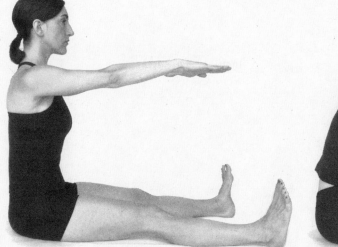

Spine Stretch Forward 1

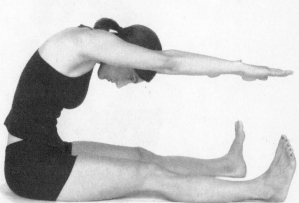

Spine Stretch Forward 2

Open Leg Rocker *(Intermediate)*

PURPOSE: **Increase balance, strengthen the abs, and massage the spine.**

Modification:

If you have neck pain, simply hold the balance with your legs extended and do not roll back (Open Leg Balance). This is a good stretch for your legs and is a challenge for your abdominal muscles to keep you balanced.

From a sitting position, pull your knees in to your chest and grab onto the top of your ankles with each hand. Lift your feet off the ground and keep your balance. Engage your abdominal muscles and straighten your knees as you extend your legs up and out about shoulder width, bringing your legs straight into a "V" position, and balance.

Inhale. Engage your abs, bring your chin toward your chest, and roll your body back, taking your legs overhead, being careful not to roll onto your neck. Using your abdominal muscles—not momentum or your arms—roll back up and balance at the top in the "V" position. Exhale. Repeat six times.

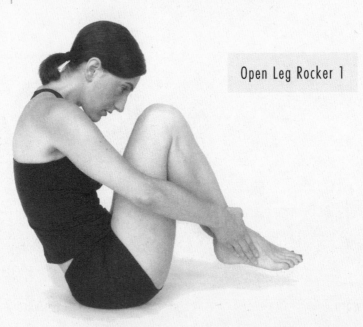

Open Leg Rocker 1

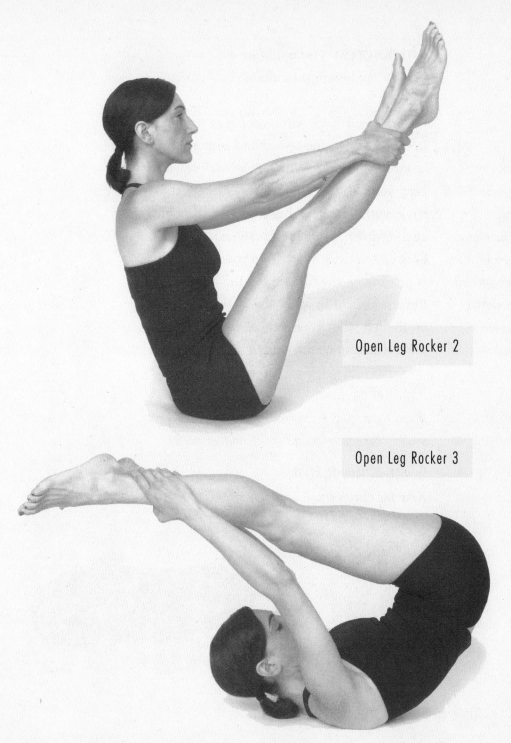

Open Leg Rocker 2

Open Leg Rocker 3

Corkscrew *(Intermediate)*
PURPOSE: Strengthen the abs.

Variation:
As you become stronger, start lifting the first four vertebrae (your butt and lower back) off the mat as the legs return to center.

Lie on your back, with your legs extended straight up to the ceiling and your arms relaxed by your sides. With feet in Pilates stance, keep your legs together as you make a small circle with your legs, beginning on the right, circling down and around to the left, and then back up to center. Work from your abs to keep your back on the mat during the movement. Reverse the direction of the circle, beginning on the left side. Repeat three times, alternating the direction each time.

Modification:
If you have lower back pain, place your hands under your buttocks and make smaller circles.

C-Section Modification:
Keep the circles small until you are completely healed.

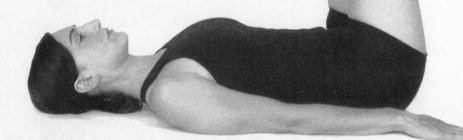

Corkscrew (Intermediate) 1

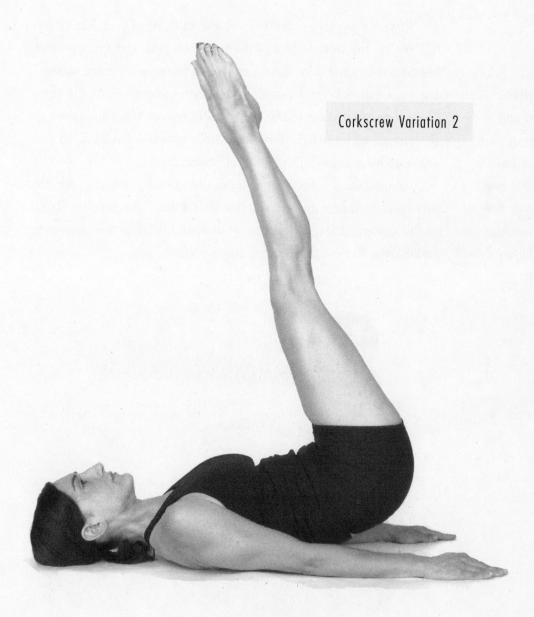

Corkscrew Variation 2

Saw *(Intermediate)*

PURPOSE: **Trim the waistline, and stretch the back and legs.**

Sit with your legs extended straight in front of you, heels resting on the outer edges of the mat. Lift your arms to shoulder height out to your sides. Inhale as you lift from your center, squeezing your buttocks and pressing your sitting bones into the mat. Twist from your waist to the right, reaching your left hand down to the outside of your right foot. Your right arm reaches back, so you are stretching in both directions. No bouncing!

Exhale the air out of your lungs completely, keeping your abs lifted and your hips anchored to the mat. Inhale as you roll up back to the center, getting taller from your waist. Twist to the other side and exhale. Repeat three times on each side.

Modification:

If you are stiff in the legs or lower back, bend your knees slightly. You may also sit on a firm pillow so your hips are slightly higher than your feet.

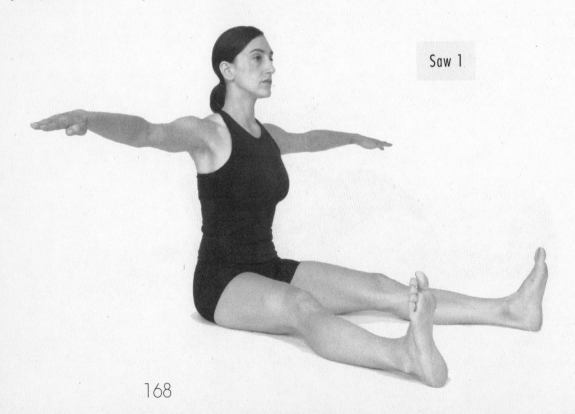

Saw 1

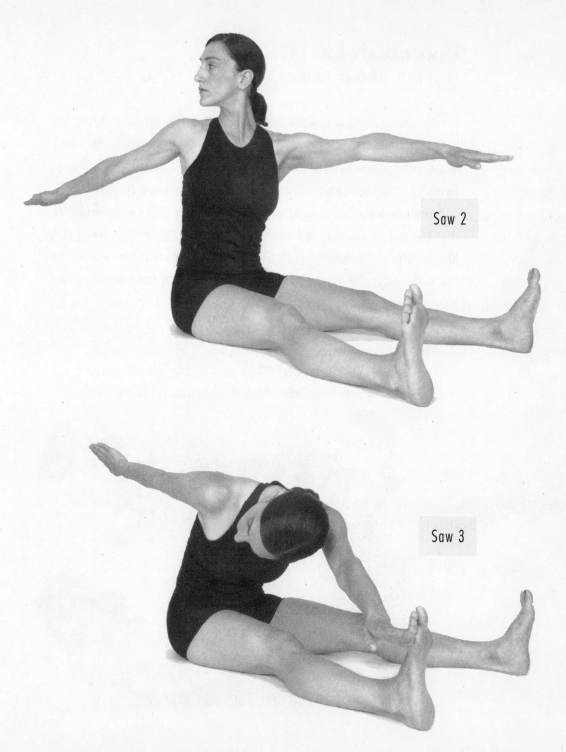

Saw 2

Saw 3

Upper Body Lift *(Advanced)*

PURPOSE: Strengthen the upper back.

Lie on your stomach with legs together and your face down on the mat. Place your palms down next to your shoulders and bend your elbows so that your arms rest alongside your body. Keeping your shoulder blades reaching down your back and abdominal muscles lifted, gently raise your upper body and hands off the mat a few inches and hold for five counts. Do not use your hands to press yourself off the mat. Slowly release. Remember to reach through the top of your head, lengthening your body as opposed to lifting your head up.

Modification:

This exercise may be uncomfortable at first if your breasts are sore or engorged or if you have lower back pain. If that is the case, skip it for now.

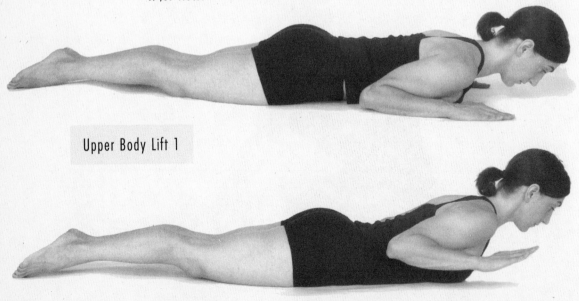

Upper Body Lift 1

Upper Body Lift 2

Neck Roll *(Intermediate)*

PURPOSE: **Strengthen the back and strengthen and stretch the neck.**

Lie on your stomach with your legs together and your face down on the mat. Place your palms down under your shoulders and bend your arms close to the body, elbows back. "Lift" your abdominal muscles (as though you are lifting your belly button) to support your lower back. Pressing into the mat with hands and forearms, push your chest off the mat, pulling your shoulder blades down to lengthen the back of your neck. Turn and look to one side, roll your chin down to your chest, then look to the other side. Reverse. Do this slowly. It is a relaxing stretch for your neck. Repeat on each side.

Modification:

This exercise may be uncomfortable at first if your breasts are sore or engorged or if you have lower back pain. If that is the case, skip it for now. When you are feeling stronger, begin the exercise with forearms into the mat. You can progress to the whole exercise later.

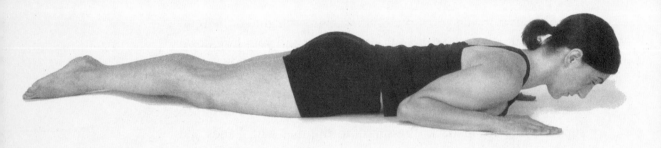

Neck Roll 1

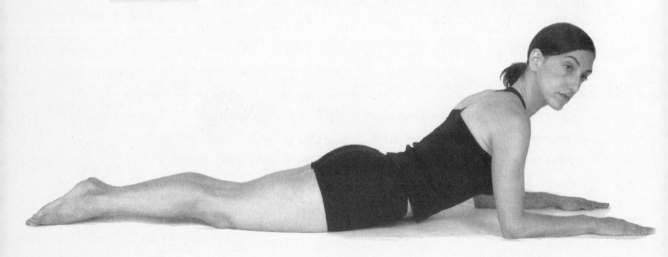

Neck Roll 2

Supermom *(Advanced)*

PURPOSE: **Strengthen the upper and lower back.**

Lie on your stomach with your arms reaching straight out in front of you. Lift your abdominal muscles, then your arms and feet a couple of inches off the floor and hold for five counts. Release. Repeat three times. Do the Spine Stretch Release (page 34) to relax your lower back.

Modification:

If you have soreness in your lower back, leave this exercise out until you become stronger.

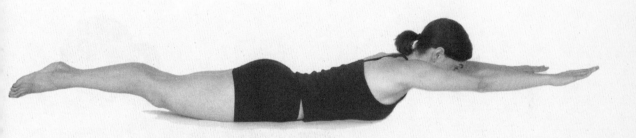

Supermom

Single Leg Kick *(Intermediate)*

PURPOSE: Stretch and strengthen the back of the legs, and strengthen the arms, chest, and buttocks.

Lie on your stomach with legs together. Prop your upper body up on your forearms; your elbows should be pointed slightly outward and your hands should be gathered in a fist directly in front of your body. Lift your abdominal muscles, chest, and head, keeping your neck long by reaching through the top of your head. Kick your buttocks two times quickly with your right leg, then with the left leg. Keep squeezing your inner thighs together.

Repeat five times, alternating legs.

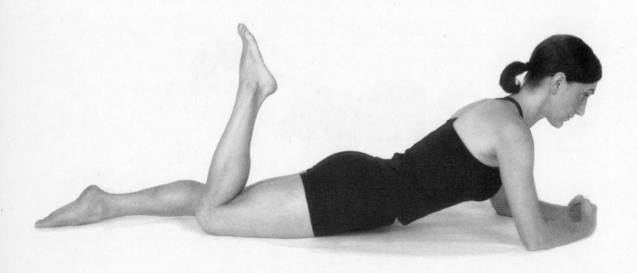

Single Leg Kick (Intermediate)

Double Leg Kick *(Intermediate)*

PURPOSE: **Stretch the chest and back, and work the legs and buttocks.**

Lie on your stomach, legs together, with one side of your face down on the mat. Bend your arms behind your back, clasping hands between your shoulder blades, with your elbows touching the mat. Kick your buttocks three times with both legs together.

After the third kick, engage your abs and straighten your legs until your toes touch the mat. Lift your upper body off the mat, opening your chest and reaching your hands straight back toward your feet. Repeat four times, alternating the direction of your head on the mat each time. Do the Spine Stretch Release (page 34) to relax the lower back.

Modification:

If you have lower back pain, leave this exercise out.

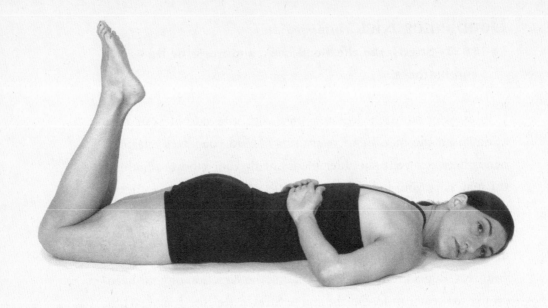

Double Leg Kick 1

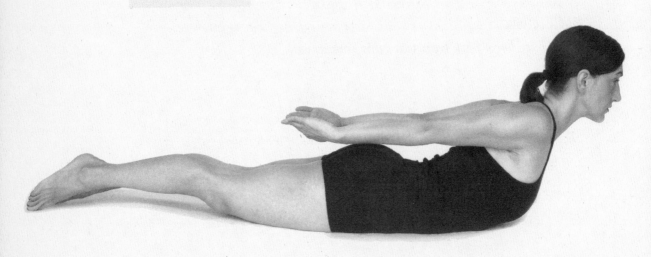

Double Leg Kick 2

176

Neck Pull *(Intermediate)*

PURPOSE: **Strengthen the abs and back for improved posture, and stretch the back of the legs.**

Lie on your back with your hands behind the base of your head and your elbows open to the sides. Keep your legs long and place your feet hip-width apart and flexed. Inhale, raise your head, bringing your chin to your chest. Begin rolling up by pulling in the upper abdominal muscles. Lift your shoulders, then the upper body, rolling all the way up, and bend forward over your legs. Exhale, bringing your head toward your knees, keeping your abs lifted in and up.

Inhale as you roll up your spine to a sitting position, maintaining elbows open to the sides with your shoulders relaxed. Sit up with a long neck and a straight spine. Start to roll back by pulling your abdominal muscles in to slide your tailbone under you and toward your flexed feet. Use your abs to push your spine into the mat all the way down, one vertebra at a time, exhaling. Repeat five times.

Modification:

If you are unable to roll up with straight legs, bend your knees slightly. If you are having difficulty rolling up at all, try it with your feet under a chair.

C-Section Modification:

Leave this exercise out until you are completely healed.

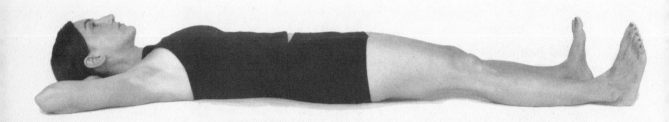

Neck Pull 1

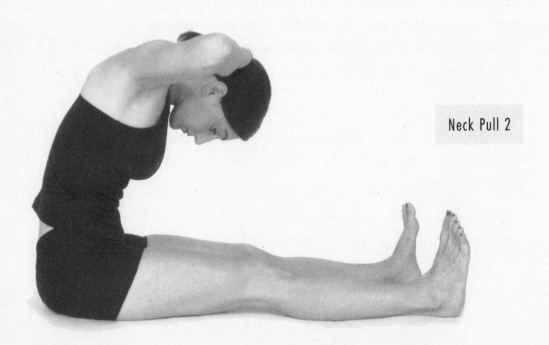

Neck Pull 2

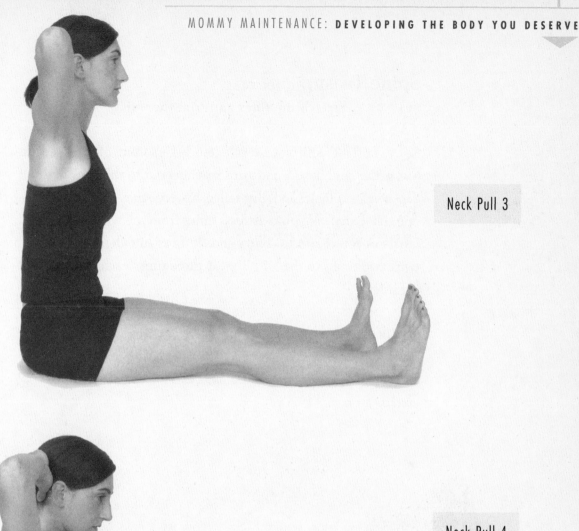

Neck Pull 3

Neck Pull 4

Spine Twist *(Advanced)*

PURPOSE: Stretch the sides and trim the waist.

Sit upright with your legs extended in front of you, feet to-gether and flexed, and arms reaching out to the sides at shoulder height. Inhale and lift taller by engaging your abdominal muscles. Exhale as you twist two times from the waist to the right. Inhale as you return to center and sit up even taller. Exhale as you twist two times to the left. Repeat three times each side, alternating sides.

Modification:

If you have trouble sitting up tall because of tight hips, keep your knees soft in the beginning. If you have lower back pain, skip this exercise for now.

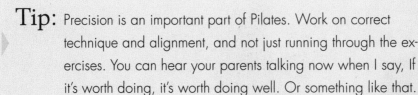

Tip: Precision is an important part of Pilates. Work on correct technique and alignment, and not just running through the exercises. You can hear your parents talking now when I say, If it's worth doing, it's worth doing well. Or something like that.

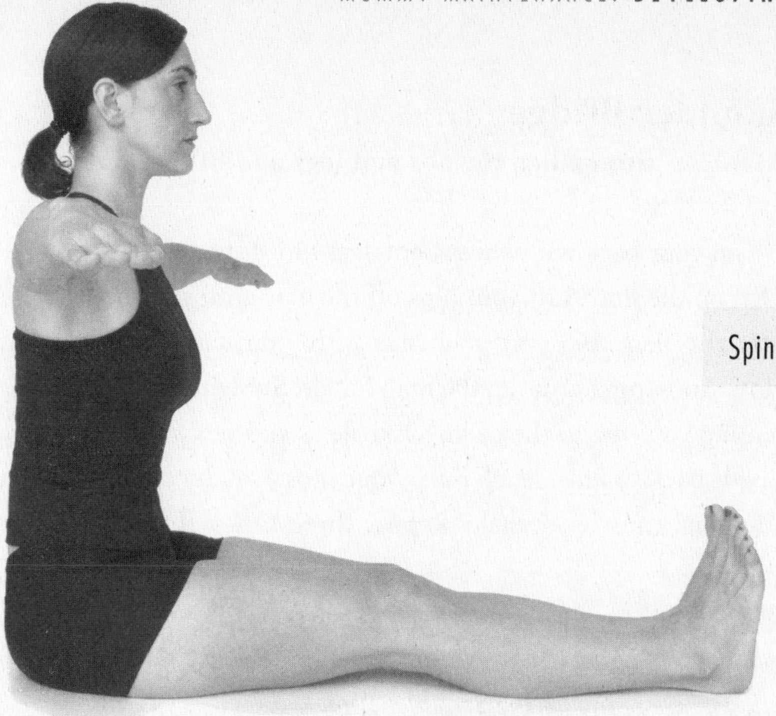

Spine Twist 1

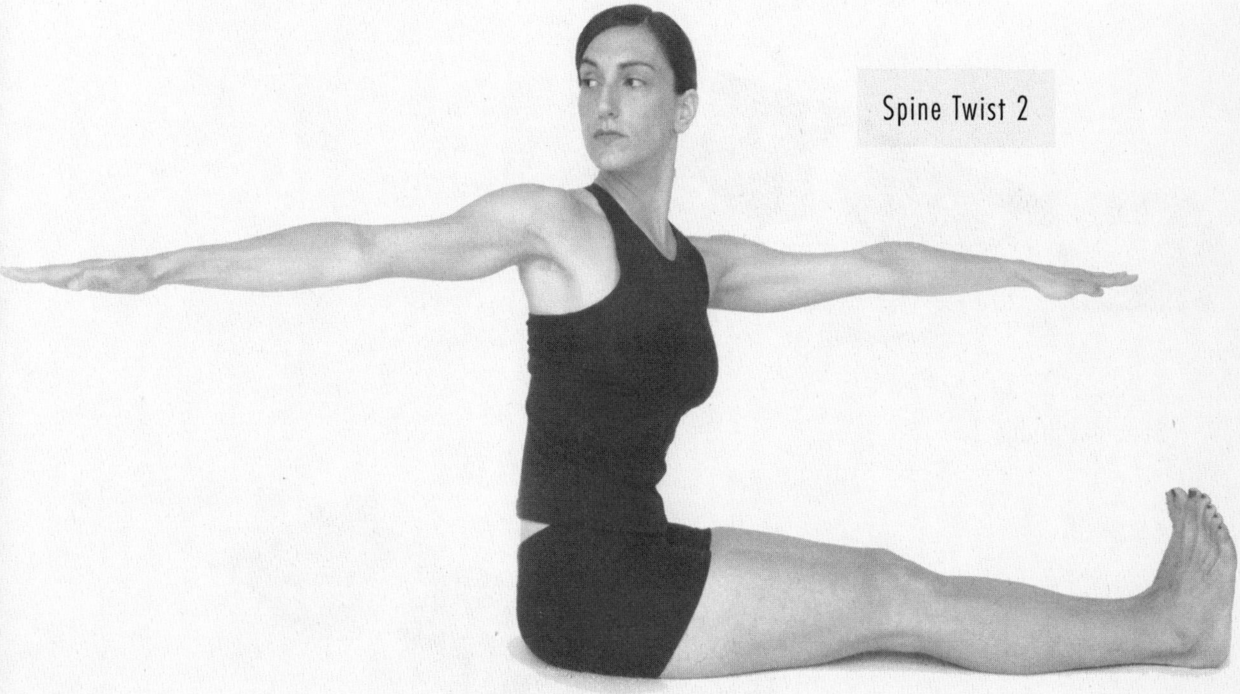

Spine Twist 2

Shoulder Bridge *(Advanced)*

PURPOSE: Strengthen the abs and legs and lift the buttocks.

Lie on your back with knees bent, legs hip-distance apart, and feet flat on the floor. Lift your hips off the mat until your body makes a straight plane. Support your hips with your hands, keeping your elbows and upper arms on the mat. Inhale. Straighten your right leg, pointing your toe to the ceiling. Exhale as you flex your foot as you bring it back to knee level. Keep your hips even by tightening your abdominal muscles. Exhale. Repeat three times, then switch legs.

Variation:
Do this exercise with your arms at your sides, relying on your abs to support the body.

Modification:
If you find this exercise too challenging, do the Pelvic Curl (page 20) until you are ready for the Shoulder Bridge.

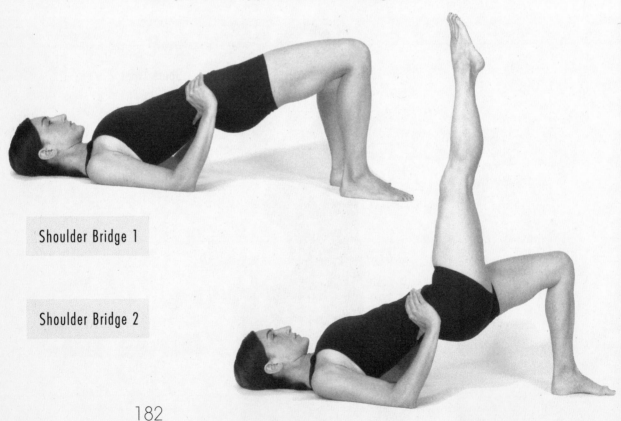

Shoulder Bridge 1

Shoulder Bridge 2

Side Kick Series

Lie on your side, lining up your back with the edge of your mat. Rest your head on your hand, with the other hand on the mat in front of your stomach. Bring your legs in front of you at a 45-degree angle (home position). Engage your abdominal muscles to stabilize the upper body, with the hips stacked on top of each other throughout the exercises. Keep your leg movements flowing and smooth. Do the full series on one side, then the Transition/Leg Beats (page 191), then switch to the other side.

FRONT/BACK *(Intermediate)*
PURPOSE: **Lengthen and tone the legs, hips, and buttocks.**

With both legs straight, lift the top leg to hip height. Slightly rotate the leg out from the hip (with knee turned toward the ceiling), keeping your leg hip height throughout the exercise. Engage your abdominal muscles and kick your leg to the front with energy. Stretch the leg long on the back kick. Repeat five to ten times.

Variation:
Bring your top hand behind your head.

Modification:
For a tired neck, place your head on your outstretched arm.

C-Section Modification:
Keep your leg movements small and controlled until you are completely pain-free around your stitches.

▶▶▶▶

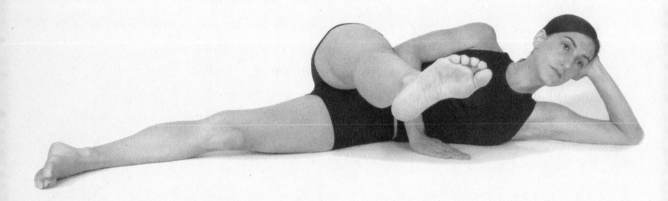

Front/Back 1

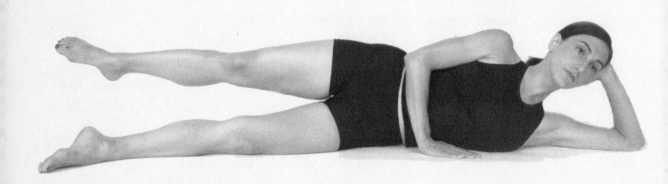

Front/Back 2

UP/DOWN *(Intermediate)*
PURPOSE: **Lengthen the legs and slim the hips, buttocks, and thighs.**

Kick your top leg up to the ceiling with energy. Lengthen your leg from the hip as you lower it to home position, resisting gravity with your inner thigh. Repeat five times.

Modification:
For a tired neck, place your head on your outstretched arm.

C-Section Modification:
Keep your leg movements small and controlled until you are completely pain-free around your stitches.

Variation:
Bring your top hand behind your head.

Up/Down

SMALL CIRCLES *(Intermediate)*
PURPOSE: Work the hips and outer thighs.

Starting with your top leg at hip height and slightly turned out, make small circles with your whole leg, not just the foot. Lengthen the leg out of the hip. Repeat five times, then reverse the circles.

Variation:

Bring your top hand behind your head.

Modification:

For a tired neck, place your head on your outstretched arm.

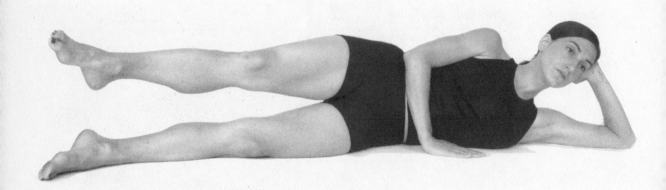

Small Circles (Intermediate)

BICYCLE *(Advanced)*

PURPOSE: **Strengthen and stretch the hips, buttocks, and legs.**

Lift your top leg up to hip height. Kick your leg forward, bend your knee, take your bent leg back, then extend it long to home position. Extend your leg long in back and feel a good stretch. Repeat three times, then reverse the movement and bicycle backward.

Variation:
Bring your top hand behind your head.

Modification:
For a tired neck, place your head on an outstretched arm.

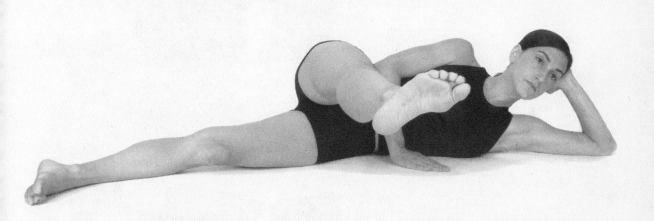

Bicycle (Advanced) 1

▶▶▶▶

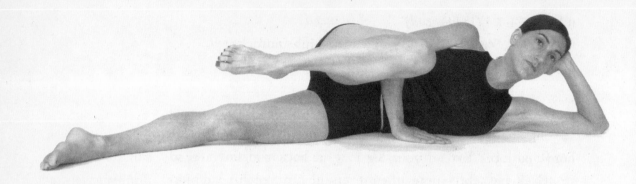

Bicycle 2

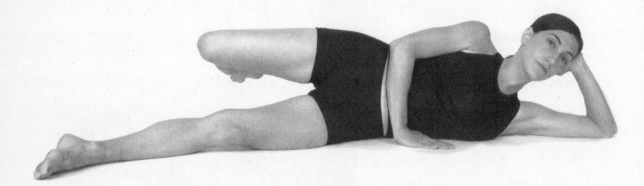

Bicycle 3

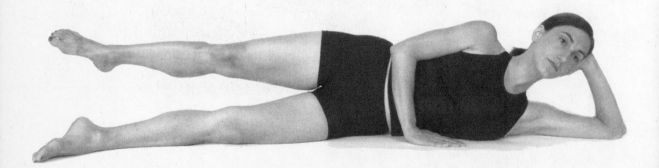

Bicycle 4

INNER THIGH LIFT *(Advanced)*

PURPOSE: **Work the inner and outer thighs and stretch the hips.**

Bend your top leg so the knee is pointed toward the ceiling and place your foot on the floor directly in front of your bottom leg (thigh). Hold on to your ankle. Lift the bottom leg from the inner thigh and reach your leg long from the hip. Stabilize your hips by engaging your abdominal muscles so your hips do not roll back. Make big circles five times in one direction, then reverse.

Modification:

If you have knee pain, leave this exercise out. For a tired neck, place your head on your outstretched arm.

Variation:

Bring your top hand behind your head.

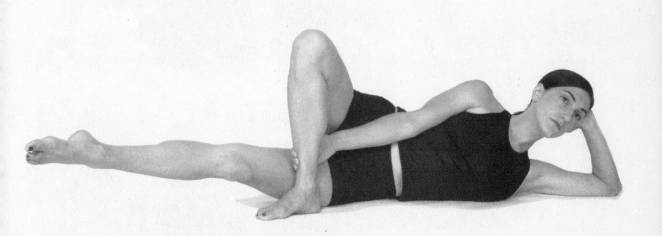

Inner Thigh Lift

189

DOUBLE LEG LIFT *(Advanced)*

PURPOSE: Strengthen the oblique muscles and work the inner and outer thighs.

Variation:

On the third repetition, keep the top leg up as you lower and lift the bottom leg ten times. Or if you find this too challenging, simply hold your legs together for ten counts.

With your inner thighs pressed together, engage your abdominal muscles to stabilize your body and lift your legs 2–5 inches off the ground. Hold for three counts, then lower your legs. Repeat three times.

Modification:

For a tired neck, place your head on your outstretched arm.

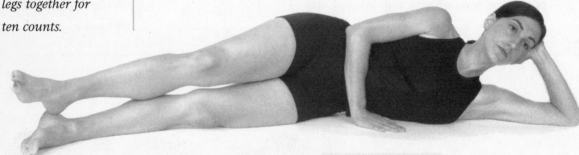

Double Leg Lift 1

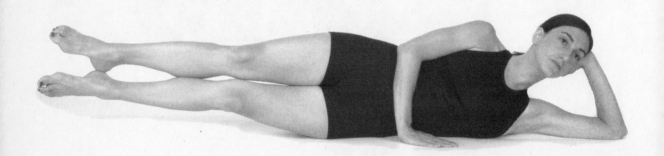

Double Leg Lift 2

TRANSITION/LEG BEATS *(Intermediate)*

PURPOSE: **Strengthen the lower back, inner and outer thighs, and butt.**

Lie on your stomach, with your forehead resting on the back of your hands and your elbows pointed out to the sides. Relax your shoulders and lift your belly off the mat to support your lower back. With your legs straight and feet in Pilates stance, lift your legs (and knees) off the mat and beat your inner thighs together. Repeat three sets of ten repetitions. When finished with the Leg Beats, turn on to your other side and repeat the Side Kick Series.

Variation:

Relaxing your upper body, bend your knees and lift them off the mat, bringing your heels toward your buttocks. This is a great exercise to "lift" your butt. Hold for five counts, then release. Repeat three times.

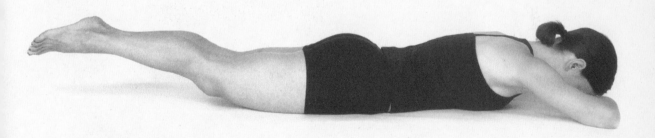

Transition/Leg Beats

191

Teaser *(Intermediate)*
PURPOSE: **Strengthen the abs and improve balance.**

Lie on your back with your arms by your ears, reaching toward the ceiling. Lift your legs to a 45-degree angle, keeping your entire back on the mat. Bring your head up and chin to chest and stretch your fingers to the sky. Inhale and roll up to reach for your toes. Balance on your sitting bones, holding the position and lifting your stomach and lower back. Keep reaching through your fingertips for your toes and exhale as you roll back down to the floor with control, keeping your legs at a 45-degree angle. Repeat three times.

Modification/C-Section Modification:
If you have difficulty holding your feet up, try bending the knees slightly, but be sure to keep your toes higher than the knees. You may also practice with your knees bent and feet on the floor, then roll up to reach for the ceiling and roll back with control.

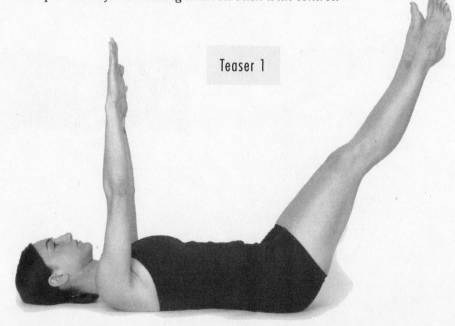

Teaser 1

192

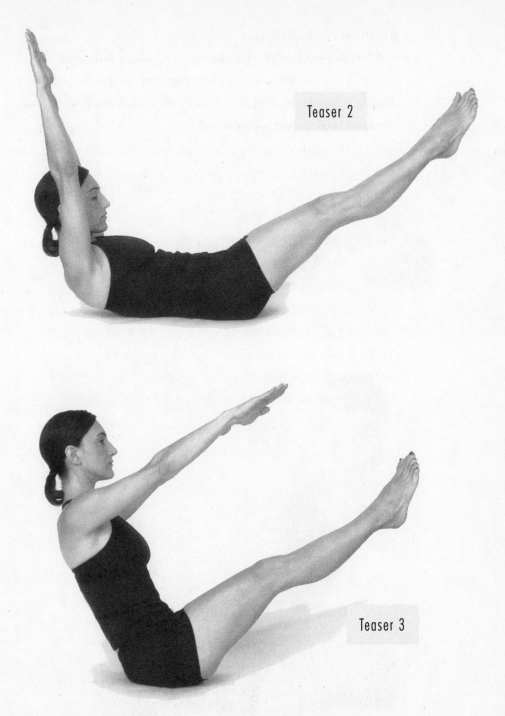

Teaser 2

Teaser 3

Variation:

Lie flat on your back with arms extended above your head. Inhale and pull in your abs to roll up, bringing arms and legs up together. Reach for your toes. Then reach your arms for the ceiling and roll the whole body down with control.

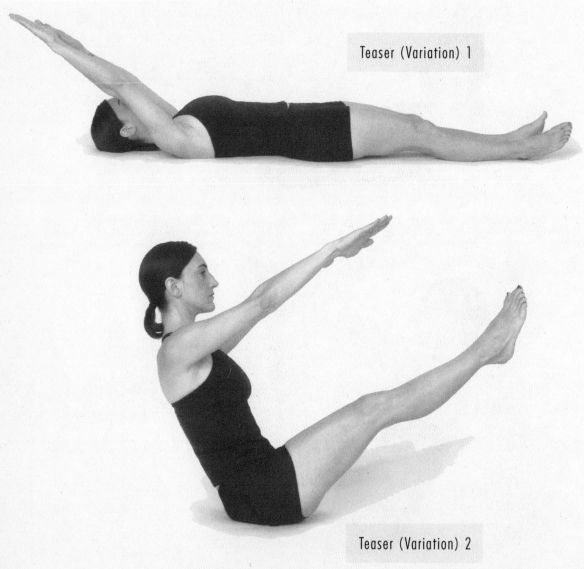

Teaser (Variation) 1

Teaser (Variation) 2

194

The Bumster *(Advanced)*

PURPOSE: **Trim the hips and waist and strengthen the abs.**

Sit upright with your legs extended in front of you and your arms bent at a 90-degree angle by your sides. Sit up tall by pulling your abdominal muscles in and lift one butt cheek off the floor and move that hip forward. Then lift the other hip and move it forward. Your arms should move naturally with you, as though you are running. Keep alternating sides and move forward for ten steps. Then reverse your direction and move backward. Repeat three to five times.

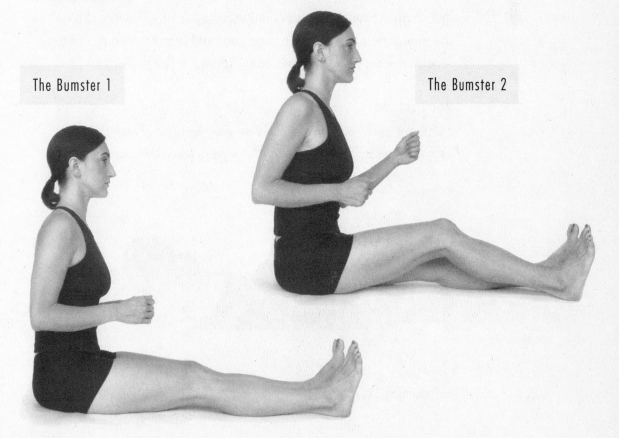

The Bumster 1

The Bumster 2

Swimming *(Advanced)*

PURPOSE: Strengthen the abs and strengthen and stretch the back.

Lying on your stomach, stretch your arms out in front of you with your legs long behind you. Raise your left arm and right leg and lift your head. Begin to alternately kick your legs up and down as you pump alternate arms up and down. Keep the abdominal muscles lifting off the mat while on your stomach to support your lower back. This will also stabilize your body so that only your arms and legs move freely. Breathe to a count of five, inhaling for five counts through the nose and exhaling for five counts through the mouth, while you pump your arms and legs. Do two sets of ten repetitions. Sit back in Spine Stretch Release (page 34).

Modification:

For a sore neck, rest your forehead on your hands and kick the legs as stated above. If you have lower back pain, leave this exercise out.

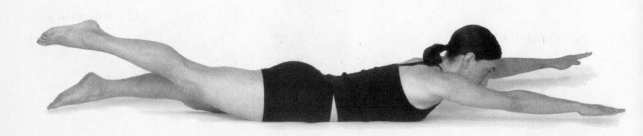

Swimming (Advanced)

> **Tip:** Do the Spine Stretch Release (page 34) after doing exercises on your stomach to release tension in your lower back.

Plank *(Advanced)*
PURPOSE: Strengthen the abs and back.

Begin on your hands and knees with your wrists lined up directly under your shoulders and your feet together. Tuck your toes under, engage your abdominal muscles, and press yourself up to a plank position (similar to a push-up position), with your feet in Pilates stance. Maintain a straight line from head to toes by pulling your shoulder blades down your back, lifting your abs, contracting your buttocks, squeezing your thighs together, and reaching your tailbone toward your heels. Hold for ten counts. Sit back in Spine Stretch Release (page 34), then repeat.

Modification:
If this is too challenging at first, do the exercise on your forearms, with your elbows directly under your shoulders.

Variation:
If you are feeling super strong, lift one leg and extend it out behind you and hold the position for five counts. Then switch legs.

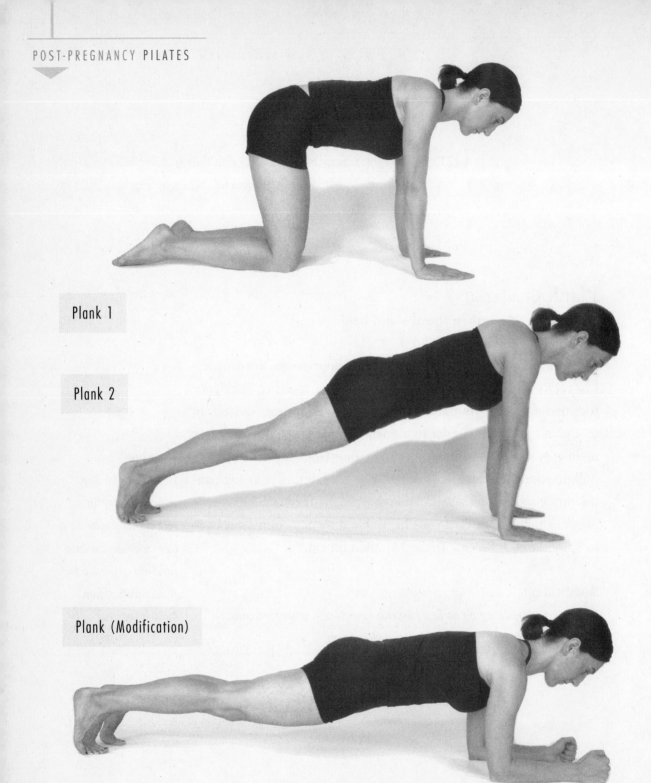

Plank 1

Plank 2

Plank (Modification)

198

Side Plank *(Advanced)*

PURPOSE: Strengthen the obliques and improve balance.

Lie on one side with your upper body propped on your elbow, which should be bent directly below your shoulder. Cross your top foot over the bottom. Your top arm rests on your side. Lift your hips off the mat by engaging your obliques so that your body forms a straight line. Hold for ten counts. Release gently to the floor. Repeat two times. Then turn on to your other side and repeat.

Variation:

When you are stronger, perform the Side Plank on your hand (instead of your forearm) and reach your top arm above your head, lined up with your ear.

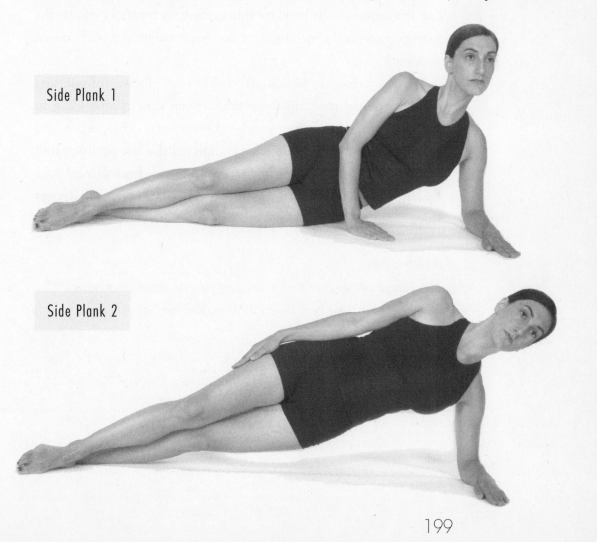

Side Plank 1

Side Plank 2

Push-up *(Advanced)*

PURPOSE: **Strengthen the upper back, chest, and arms.**

Stand with your feet in Pilates stance and arms raised above your head. Bring your chin to chest, engage your abdominal muscles and begin to roll down your spine until your hands reach the floor. With straight legs, walk your hands forward on the mat until your wrists are directly below your shoulders and your body is in a straight line (like the Plank, page 197). Maintain this straight line throughout your body by squeezing your buttocks and thighs together, keeping your abs tight and your shoulder blades down your back.

Bend your arms backward so that your elbows are pointing behind you and push up three times. Keep your elbows close to your ribs and inhale when you bend your arms, exhale when you raise your body. When you have completed the last push-up, pull your abs in to lift your hips and walk your hands back toward your feet. Roll up slowly to standing, lifting your arms overhead. Repeat three times.

Modification:

If regular Push-ups are too challenging for you, bring your knees down to the mat for bent-knee Push-ups. You may also do them against the wall (page 121).

Push-up 1

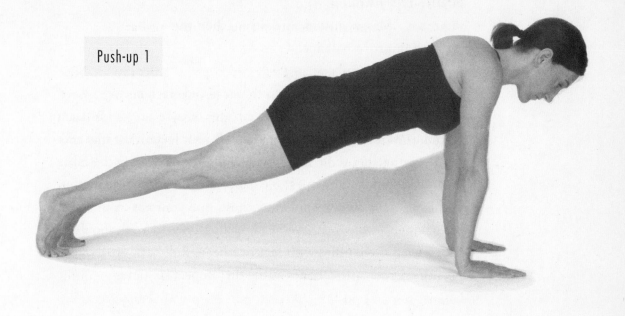

Push-up 2

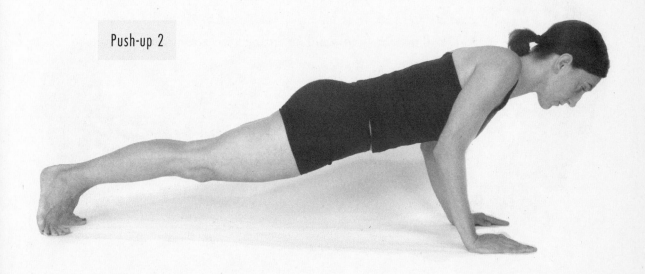

Seal *(Intermediate)*

PURPOSE: Massage the spine, strengthen the abs, and improve balance.

Sitting up, bend your knees to the sides and reach between your legs and under your feet to grab the outside of your ankles. Keep the insides of your feet together. Lift your feet off the mat and clap them together three times by opening your legs from the hips. Use your abdominal muscles to balance on your sitting bones. Inhale. Bring your chin toward your chest, pull your abs in, and roll back, bringing your feet overhead, rolling only to your shoulder blades. Clap three times with feet overhead. Roll back up. Exhale. Balance on your sitting bones at the top. Repeat six times.

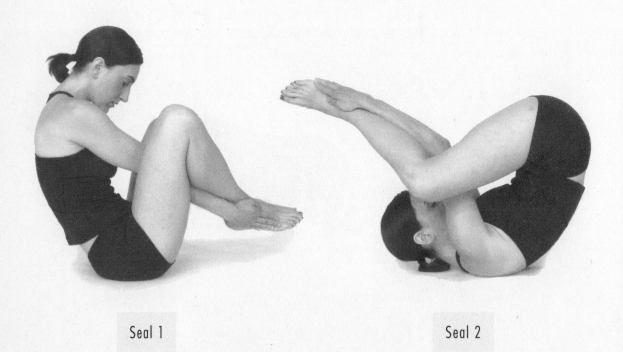

Seal 1

Seal 2

8

Time-Saving Mini Programs:
Crib Notes for the Busy Mom

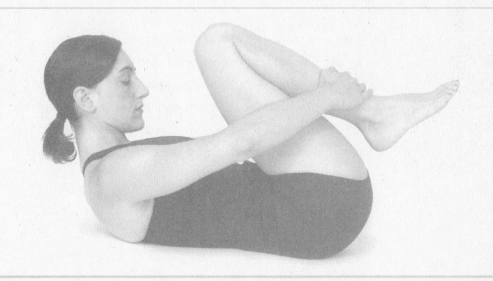

We all become proficient multitaskers as mothers. With everything we must accomplish during the course of the day, efficiency is the name of the game. That is also true of Pilates—it is the most time-effective exercise method in that the movements are focused and require very few repetitions.

Pilates is a complete program that combines strengthening and stretching for every part of the body. Given the time constraints of new mothers, I have put together some mini programs that include exercises for the whole body, but that are more time efficient than trying to fit in the whole routine and having to stop in the middle because of baby interruptions. These programs, presuming you are now familiar with the exercises, should take no longer than 15–20 minutes.

Tip: Take time at the end of the weekend to schedule time for exercise in the upcoming week. Don't give up or be discouraged by what your scale says. Focus on your long-term health. You will see results and you will be pleased. All bodies are not created equal, and sometimes genetics do not work in our favor and it takes a little longer to fit into your pre-baby clothes.

TIME-SAVER 1

1 • Hundred

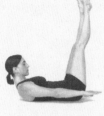

2 • Roll Back

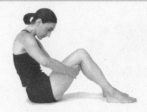

3 • Pelvic Curl

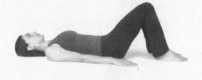

4 • Single Leg Stretch

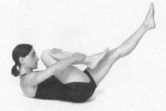

5 • Double Leg Stretch

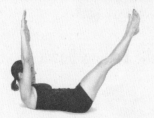

6 • Spine Stretch Forward

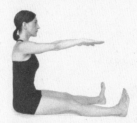

7 • Upper Body Lift

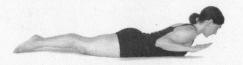

8 • Neck Roll

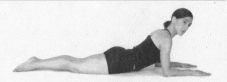

TIME-SAVER 1

9 • Spine Stretch Release

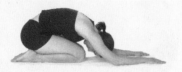

10 • Teaser

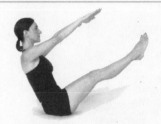

11 • Seal

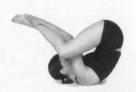

12 • Wall: Push-ups

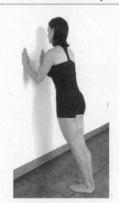

13 • Wall: Squat

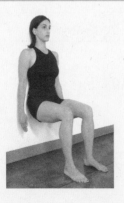

14 • Wall: Rolling Down

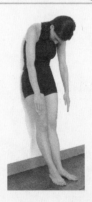

TIME-SAVER 2

1 • Hundred

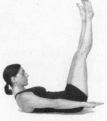

2 • Roll Up

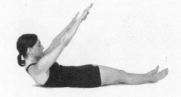

3 • Single Leg Circles

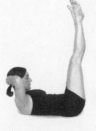

4 • Single Straight Leg

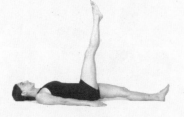

5 • Double Straight Leg

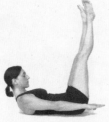

6 • Crisscross

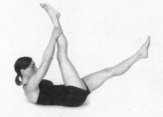

7 • Spine Stretch Forward

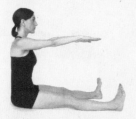

8 • Open Leg Rocker

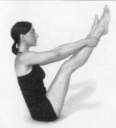

TIME-SAVER 2

9 • Supermom

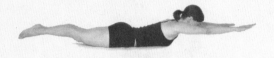

10 • Single Leg Kicks

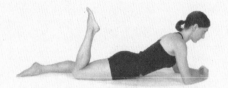

11 • Neck Pull

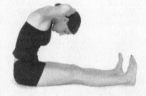

12 • Shoulder Bridge

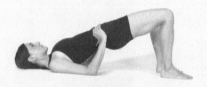

13 • Side Kicks: Front/Back

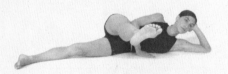

14 • Side Kicks: Up/Down

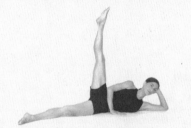

15 • Side Kicks: Small Circles

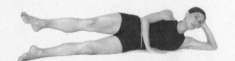

16 • Side Kicks: Beats

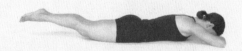

TIME-SAVER 2

17 • Seal

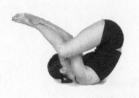

18 • Arm Weights: Biceps Curl

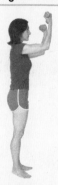

19 • Arm Weights: Zip Up

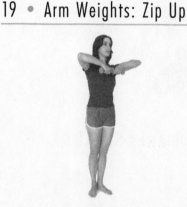

20 • Arm Weights: Shaving

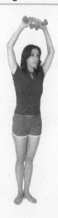

21 • Arm Weights: Lunge

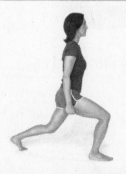

Tip: All weeks are not created equal. You will have some good days and some bad days when you can't do as much as you would like. Give yourself a break and then keep moving forward.

TIME-SAVER 3

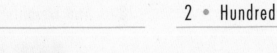

1 • Breathing

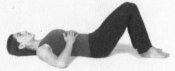

2 • Hundred

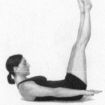

3 • Roll Up

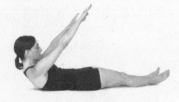

4 • Rolling Like a Ball

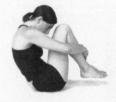

5 • Single Leg Stretch

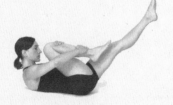

6 • Double Leg Stretch

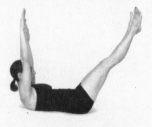

7 • Single Straight Leg

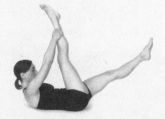

8 • Double Straight Leg

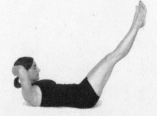

TIME-SAVER 3

9 • Spine Stretch Forward

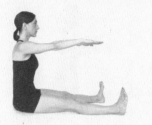

10 • Corkscrew

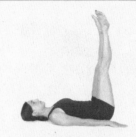

11 • Saw

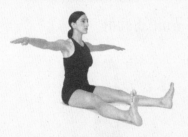

12 • Side Kicks: Front/Back

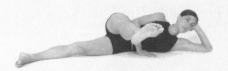

13 • Side Kick: Inner Thigh Lifts

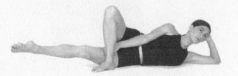

14 • Side Kick: Beats

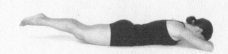

15 • Teaser

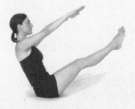

16 • Swimming

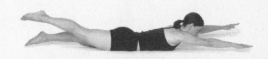

TIME-SAVER 3

17 • Plank

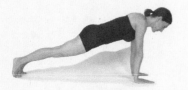

18 • Wall: Push-ups

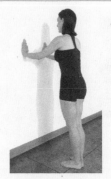

19 • Wall: Arm Circles

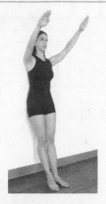

20 • Wall: Squat

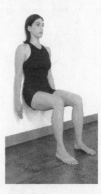

21 • Wall: Rolling Down

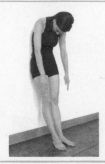

Tip: Buy workout clothes that make you feel good. You don't have to wear your stretched-out sweatpants and oversized T-shirts. It will make a difference in how you view yourself and your fitness commitment.

9

Taking It Off the Mat:
Pilates in Your Daily Life

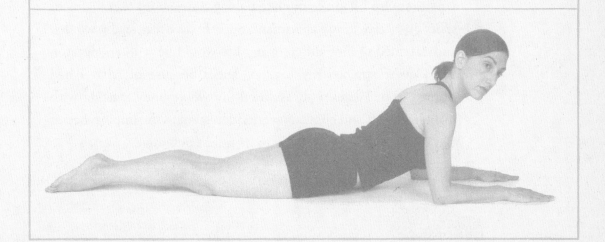

Now that you are a total pro at your Pilates routine and you understand the basic principles behind the method, you can take this knowledge out into the world and put it to practical use. Remember that using your core muscles is the key not only to performing the exercises, but also to lifting your baby, reaching for something on a high shelf, carrying heavy grocery bags, or even sitting at your desk for extended periods of time. The core muscles stabilize your movements, enable you to perform tasks more efficiently and effectively, and keep you from injuring yourself.

It is easy to forget about protecting your back. You are lifting and carrying a baby and all the extra gear needed for the baby, constantly bending over to pick things up, and generally not paying attention to yourself. Over time, this can lead to serious backaches. Use your abdominal muscles, bend your knees, avoid sudden twisting, and keep your back straight when performing all of the above-mentioned tasks.

I had the misfortune of living in a walk-up building when Ches was born, which meant I had to carry a stroller, a baby, and whatever else I had accumulated along the way up two flights of stairs every day to my apartment. Sure, I was occasionally winded and dreamed of how different my life would be with an elevator, but I never strained my back or knees because of what I had learned from Pilates. I always used my whole body, starting with my core, to lift and climb. Never underestimate the importance of the details, and use your body to its fullest potential.

Picking Up Baby

When lifting the baby from a crib or changing table (or anyplace that is slightly below waist level), be sure when bending from the waist to also bend your knees, engage your core (abdominal muscles), and use your whole body. Don't just use your arms to reach and lift.

Carrying Baby

We often find ourselves resting the baby on one hip, and it is usually the opposite hip of your dominant hand (right-handed women place the baby on their left hip) for convenience in performing other tasks. This position stresses the hip joint and can cause tightness or pain in your hip, back, or knee. An equal distribution of your weight is necessary to maintain a comfortable position. It is best to avoid resting your baby on one side. But, if you must rest the baby on one hip, be aware of your posture and only stand that way for brief periods of time. The same goes for holding the baby over one shoulder, as well as carrying the baby in a front carrier. The "correct" positions are:

◆ **The airplane hold**—a favorite of many dads—has the baby facedown with his tummy resting on your forearm and his head by the crook of your elbow. Your hands can grasp under the diaper area (a good way to know when it's changing time). This hold keeps the baby in front and you can still maintain good posture by

keeping your abs in and shoulders rolled back with
an open chest.

- ◆ **Regular front hold** has the baby facing you with his
head at your shoulder height. This is a good hold
because you can switch sides and keep your weight
equally distributed on both feet.
- ◆ **Front-facing hold** with baby facing out in front of you
is good for baby to see what is going on around him,
and you can also switch arms.

Feeding Baby

Finding a comfortable feeding and/or breastfeeding position
that suits you is challenging in the beginning. When settling in
a chair at home, make sure the arms of the chair are the correct height for holding the baby close enough to you—with his
head in the crook of your elbow and your other arm under his body
to support him—so you don't have to slouch to reach the baby. Alternatively, you can support the baby on a firm pillow. Once you
are comfortably installed in your seat, take a moment to do your
toe-to-head check:

- ◆ **Feet:** Your feet should either touch the ground while your
back is fully supported against the back of the chair or
they should be elevated so your back is supported.
- ◆ **Legs:** Your legs should be uncrossed and relaxed and if
bent, at more or less a right angle.
- ◆ **Butt:** Both butt cheeks should be seated on the chair with
weight equally distributed to both sides.

◆ **Lower back:** Your back should be fully supported against the back of the chair. A small pillow can help if necessary.

◆ **Middle back:** The middle back should be upright and supported by the chair.

◆ **Upper back/shoulders:** These also should be upright—not slouching forward—and supported by the back of the chair. To coerce your shoulders into the proper position, try to pull your shoulder blades together and down your back. This will encourage a natural upright position in the upper back and will avoid the common problem of pulling shoulders back and jutting the chest out, which compromises the support of your back.

◆ **Neck/head:** Yes, of course you can gaze lovingly into your baby's eyes while feeding, but remember to straighten your neck occasionally to avoid a cramp or stiffness that will curse you later.

◆ **Abs:** As always, continue to lengthen and lift your abdominal muscles.

Playtime

If you are sitting on the floor with the baby, position yourself so that your weight is evenly distributed on both hips and pull your abdominal muscles in and up to keep a straight spine. Avoid spending too much time sitting on your knees by changing your position periodically.

Getting Up from the Floor

If you are getting up by yourself, keep one knee bent and place your other foot on the floor. Engage your abdominal muscles and push up with your legs. Use your hands if necessary to help boost yourself up. If you are getting up and need to pick up the baby as well, get up by yourself first. Rest on one knee with the other foot planted firmly on the floor. Engage your abdominal muscles, bend from the waist, and keep a straight spine to pick up the baby with both arms. To stand from this position, hold the baby close to you and stand up using your abs and legs to push yourself up. If you need to hold on to a chair for assistance, make sure it is stable.

Household Chores

Finally, while folding laundry, cleaning, or doing other household chores, keep these rules in mind: Bend your knees, always engage your abdominal muscles (hey, they are still working, getting stronger even while doing the dishes—this is a bonus!), and keep your shoulders down and back with your chest open. And be aware of your neck, keeping it long and tension-free.

Does this seem like a lot of instructions for such mundane tasks? Perhaps, but these small adjustments will make a huge difference in your comfort level and ultimately your overall strength and posture that is worth the few seconds it takes to incorporate them into your routines.

Getting In and Out of Cars

It is very important—especially if you are carrying the baby in the car seat—to be aware of your position getting in and out of the car. Bend your knees and engage your abdominal muscles to bend over from your waist, and use your whole body to pick up the baby.

At Work

Follow these basic rules at work and you will feel and see the subtle differences from hunched over and tired to tall and energetic:

- Make sure to alternate shoulders when carrying a shoulder bag, or better yet, carry a handbag. Shoulder bags and purses tend to encourage uneven shoulders, tension in the neck, and poor posture.
- When sitting at your desk, make sure your chair is supportive and your knees are bent at a right angle and your feet touch the ground while you sit comfortably supporting your back against the chair. Sit up by pulling your stomach in, not by lifting your shoulders or leaning your elbows on your desk.
- Keep your keyboard directly in front of your body, not off to one side.
- If you talk on the phone while working on the computer, use a headset. You may feel silly, but headsets will save your neck and shoulders from future agony. And you can secretly pretend you are Madonna/Britney/Janet, or even Lily Tomlin.

Desk Exercises

To relieve pain or tension caused by being a working mom, you can perform many of the exercises and stretches in this book at your desk or in your office. Start by practicing your breathing (page 19) and doing the Tummy Tightener exercise (page 46) and Kegels (page 18). Then try out these other simple movements.

1 • Neck Circles

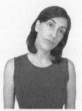

2 • Shoulder Rolls

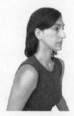

3 • Shoulder Elevation

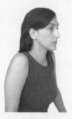

4 • Neck Exercise

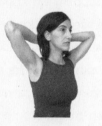

5 • Backward Arms

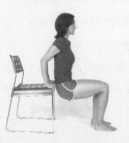

6 • Wall: Push-ups

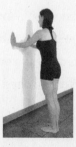

Driving

You are not a teenager anymore so that cool driving slouch has to go. Adjust your seat back and the seat cushion so that you are close enough to the steering wheel and pedals to keep your back up against the seat. Crazy traffic, a screaming baby, a bad song on the radio—no matter the stress instigator, keep your shoulders relaxed. And P.S. Don't drive and talk on the phone!

Wearing the Front Carrier or Backpack

When using a front carrier, you are almost replicating the weight load from your pregnancy; however, this time the child is heavier and the stress is more on your shoulders and neck. Adjust the straps of the carrier so that the baby is not hanging down around your waist. Engage your abdominal muscles to keep your back upright and protected. And utilize your upper back muscles (between the shoulder blades) to pull your shoulders back, working against the gravity (and baby) that pulls them down and forward. Try to avoid carrying anything else, but if you must carry groceries, etc., balance the weight in both arms.

For the backpack, make sure it fits snuggly to your back and use the waist belt to help keep it stable. It should also help to provide some lower back support (like a weight belt). Now that the excess weight is on your upper back, the tendency will be for your whole upper body to lean forward, or worse, push your hips forward, jut out your chest, and destroy your lower back. Again, avoid carrying anything but your baby in the pack and keep your abdominal muscles engaged. When you feel the baby is getting too heavy to be carried this way, don't just forge ahead and ignore the strain. It is time to put that baby in a stroller!

Pushing the Stroller

In New York City, my stroller was like my car. In fact, it was better than a car because it was easy to park, too small to accumulate trash, and enabled me to get exercise while running errands. You do not, of course, want to be hunched over the stroller or lean into it. Stand up tall and push with your whole body, not just your arms.

Standing

If you are standing for long periods of time, especially when carrying the baby, but even without him, distribute your weight evenly on both feet. You can even do your Kegels and Tummy Tighteners and no one will be the wiser.

Carrying Groceries, Car Seat, and Other Gear

Carry the car seat in front of you with both arms, being careful not to arch your back and push your hips forward. Evenly distribute the weight of the bags when you are carrying groceries. Take more trips than you would normally do—from the car to the house, up the stairs, etc. Efficiency is great but you don't want to pay for it later by being careless with your body.

CONCLUSION

My outlook on life changed so drastically after Ches was born. I became a much happier, more outgoing person due to an indescribable love for him that quietly infiltrated my whole life. I suppose it was the fatigue and the overwhelming feeling of joy at the sight of my little fuzzy guy, but during the first few weeks all I could do was stare at him and cry happy tears. I still find myself staring at him. When he becomes a teenager he will probably think I am totally embarrassing, and I will most likely be mortified by some horribly trendy haircut he insists on getting. But I will let him do his thing, as I do mine, which includes Pilates and trying to age gracefully and happily. My love for him changes and grows as he does. And he is my ultimate motivation to stay strong and healthy.

Now that you have experienced how integrating Pilates into your lifestyle makes you feel, hopefully you will be inspired to continue with the program even after you are finished with this book. What you have learned from this book you can pass along to your friends, sisters, and even your children. Whether you are a working mom, stay-at-home mom, or somewhere in between, seeing you happy and fit will motivate others to lead a healthy lifestyle. And don't forget to congratulate yourself. You are someone's mom, and you look great.

INDEX

ABOUT THE AUTHOR

◀◀◀◀ Karrie Adamany is the founder of Mommy Maintenance, a Pilates program specifically designed for new mothers to regain their fitness after pregnancy and childbirth. She is also the co-owner of The Pilates Edge Studio in New York City, and the coauthor of *The Pilates Edge: An Athlete's Guide to Strength and Performance* (Avery, 2004). Karrie is the founder of ablab®, a service that sends certified Pilates instructors to private residences and hotels. Adamany has been practicing Pilates since 1998, and was certified by Romana Kryzanowska, Master Teacher and authority on the Pilates method as taught by Joseph Pilates. She lives in New York City with her family.